Disability
Empowerment
Healthcare, Social Care, Education & Childcare

HSC TRAINING LINK

DEDICATION

This book is intended for a diverse readership committed to understanding and advancing disability empowerment. It serves as a valuable resource for educators, healthcare professionals, social workers, caregivers, policymakers, advocates and anyone interested in championing the rights and autonomy of individuals with disabilities.

Whether you are a student seeking comprehensive insights into disability empowerment or a practitioner looking to enhance your knowledge and practice, this book provides a holistic view of the principles, practices and legal frameworks that underpin the empowerment of individuals with disabilities.

It is also a valuable reference for individuals with disabilities themselves, their families and support networks, offering guidance on navigating systems, asserting rights and fostering a sense of self-determination.

With a commitment to inclusivity and empowerment, this book aims to empower readers to create more inclusive, equitable and supportive communities for individuals with disabilities.

CONTENTS

ACKNOWLEDGMENTS

The information and insights provided in this document draw upon a synthesis of various sources, including academic literature, authoritative websites and general knowledge. The content is based on a broad understanding of the topics discussed and while specific sources are not cited, the information presented is aligned with established principles and practices in the fields of disability empowerment, disability rights, healthcare, social care, education and childcare. For specific references and further reading on these topics, the following sources and domains can be consulted:

International Disability Alliance
Disability Foundation
Sense
Disability Rights UK
National Autistic Society
British Deaf Association
MIND
Mencap
UK Government

1 INTRODUCTION

In a society that values diversity and inclusivity, the concept of disability empowerment has emerged as a vital component of ensuring that individuals with disabilities are afforded equal opportunities, rights and autonomy.

This book sets out to provide a comprehensive and objective examination of disability empowerment, its principles, components and practical applications.

The Scholarly Exploration

The following chapters offer an academic exploration of disability empowerment, grounded in research, legislation and evidence-based practices.

There will be a systematic examination the core principles that underpin disability empowerment and the various components that contribute to its realisation, providing a clear and structured understanding of the subject matter.

Dissecting Disability Empowerment

Your journey begins with a thorough examination of the principles that drive disability empowerment, emphasising the importance of personalised care tailored to individual needs, preferences and goals.

We will explore the significance of informed decision-making, the role of self-determination in care planning and the critical advocacy efforts that promote equal access and rights for individuals with disabilities.

A Framework for Learning

As you progress through the chapters, you will encounter insights into the role of skill-building in fostering independence, along with the importance of nurturing a positive self-image among individuals with disabilities.

You will be provided with practical guidance on implementing disability empowerment principles in various contexts, including healthcare, education, community support services and childcare.

A Resource for Learning

This book is designed for students, professionals and researchers seeking a solid foundation in the field of disability empowerment.

It aims to equip readers with the knowledge and tools necessary to promote empowerment and inclusion for individuals with disabilities within diverse settings.

A valuable resource for those interested in understanding the principles and practices of disability empowerment, approaching the topic objectively and academically, offering a framework for critical thinking and informed decision-making in the realm of disability empowerment.

Understanding disability empowerment is not merely an academic exercise; it is a pragmatic necessity.

In a society that aspires to uphold principles of equity, inclusivity and individual rights, a comprehensive understanding of disability empowerment is vital.

Why such understanding is required requires examining the practical, social and ethical dimensions of this imperative.

Practical Imperative

At a practical level, comprehending disability empowerment is essential for service providers, caregivers, educators, policymakers and individuals with disabilities themselves.

It serves as a foundational framework upon which effective policies, programs and support services can be built.

Without such understanding, well-intentioned efforts may lack the necessary precision to address the diverse needs, preferences and goals of individuals with disabilities.

A nuanced understanding of disability empowerment can lead to the development of tailored interventions that maximise independence, self-determination and overall well-being.

Social Imperative

From a societal perspective, understanding disability empowerment is crucial for fostering an inclusive community.

It challenges the barriers and stigmas that have persisted historically and encourages active participation and contribution by individuals with disabilities.

Without this understanding, societal attitudes may inadvertently perpetuate stereotypes, discrimination and exclusion, hindering the full integration of individuals with disabilities into all facets of community life.

A society that values diversity and recognises the potential of every individual is contingent upon a collective understanding of disability empowerment.

From a societal perspective, an inclusive community is crucial for several reasons:

1. **Promotion of Diversity and Equality:**

- An inclusive community values and celebrates diversity in all its forms, including but not limited to disability.

- It recognises that every individual, regardless of their background or abilities, has a unique contribution to make.

- This promotes equality by ensuring that no one is excluded or marginalised based on their differences.

2. **Social Cohesion:**

- Inclusive communities foster a sense of belonging and 'connectedness' among all members.

- When individuals with disabilities are included and treated as equals, it strengthens social bonds and reduces the likelihood of social isolation.

- This sense of cohesion benefits the entire community by creating a more harmonious and supportive environment.

3. **Maximising Human Potential:**

- By embracing inclusivity, communities tap into the full spectrum of human potential.

- This means that individuals with disabilities are

given the opportunity to showcase their talents, skills and abilities, contributing to the enrichment and advancement of society as a whole.

4. **Economic Growth:**

- Inclusive communities recognise that individuals with disabilities can be valuable contributors to the workforce and the economy.

- When everyone has access to employment opportunities and can participate in economic activities, it leads to greater economic growth and stability.

5. **Fulfilment of Legal and Ethical Obligations:**

- Many countries have enacted legislation to promote inclusivity and protect the rights of individuals with disabilities.

- An inclusive community ensures compliance with these legal and ethical obligations, preventing discrimination and upholding human rights principles.

6. **Improved Quality of Life:**

- Inclusive communities prioritise accessibility, which benefits everyone, not just individuals with disabilities.

- This includes accessible public spaces, transportation, education and healthcare.

- Such improvements enhance the overall quality of life for all community members.

7. **Positive Social Values:**

- Inclusivity helps instil positive social values such as empathy, compassion and respect.

- When children and adults interact with individuals with disabilities in inclusive settings, it promotes understanding and challenges stereotypes, leading to a more compassionate and accepting society.

8. **Social and Cultural Enrichment:**

- Diversity within a community enriches its social and cultural fabric.

- Inclusive communities often host a variety of cultural events, share different traditions and embrace a wide range of perspectives.

- This cultural richness fosters a vibrant and dynamic community life.

9. **Resilience and Preparedness:**

- Inclusive communities tend to be more resilient and better prepared to address crises or emergencies.

- When individuals with disabilities are integrated into disaster preparedness and response plans, it ensures that the needs of all community members are considered.

10. **Future Sustainability:**

- As societies evolve, an inclusive mindset becomes increasingly relevant.

- An ageing population, for example, may experience disability-related challenges, making inclusive practices essential for future sustainability.

Ethical Imperative

On an ethical note, understanding disability empowerment is fundamental to upholding the principles of human rights and social justice.

It acknowledges the rights of individuals with disabilities to lead lives that are not limited by their conditions and advocates for equitable access to opportunities and resources.

Failure to recognise disability empowerment can result in ethical violations, as individuals with disabilities may be denied their right to make choices, assert their preferences and live independently.

Understanding this concept is integral to ensuring ethical conduct and adherence to the principles of autonomy and dignity.

From an ethical perspective, the principles of human rights and social justice are foundational concepts that guide our understanding of fairness, equity and the treatment of individuals within society.

These principles are intrinsically linked and play a vital role in promoting a just and humane society.

Here's an explanation of each principle:

1. Human Rights:

Definition: Human rights are fundamental, inalienable entitlements and protections that every individual possesses simply by virtue of being human. They are universal, indivisible and inherent to all individuals, regardless of their nationality, race, gender, religion or other characteristics.

Key Aspects of Human Rights:

- **Universality:** Human rights apply to all individuals, without discrimination. They are not subject to geographical or cultural variations.

- **Inalienability:** Human rights cannot be taken away, transferred or forfeited. They are inherent to every person from birth to death.

- **Indivisibility:** Human rights are interconnected and interdependent. They encompass civil, political, economic, social and cultural rights.

- **Equality and Non-Discrimination:** Human rights demand that all individuals are treated with equal dignity and worth and discrimination on any grounds is prohibited.

- **Protection and Accountability:** Governments and institutions are responsible for respecting, protecting and fulfilling human rights. There are mechanisms, both national and international, to hold violators accountable.

2. Social Justice:

Definition: Social justice is the concept of ensuring that every member of society has equitable access to opportunities, resources and benefits. It seeks to rectify existing inequalities and address systemic injustices.

Key Aspects of Social Justice:

- **Equity:** Social justice promotes fairness and aims to eliminate disparities in areas such as wealth, education, employment and healthcare. It recognises that people have different needs and may require different levels of support to achieve equality.

- **Redistribution:** To achieve social justice, resources and opportunities may need to be redistributed to ensure that marginalised or disadvantaged groups have equal access to societal benefits.

- **Participation and Inclusion:** Social justice encourages the full participation and inclusion of all individuals in society's decision-making processes, regardless of their background or abilities.

- **Human Dignity:** Central to social justice is the respect for human dignity. It recognises the intrinsic worth of every individual and seeks to uphold their rights and well-being.

- **Systemic Change:** Achieving social justice often requires systemic changes in laws, policies and institutions to remove barriers and promote equality.

The Interplay of Human Rights and Social Justice:

Human rights and social justice are intertwined. Human rights provide the ethical foundation for social justice efforts. Social justice, in turn, serves as a practical mechanism for realising and protecting human rights. When society pursues social justice, it works towards ensuring that individuals can fully exercise their human rights.

For example, addressing issues such as discrimination, poverty and unequal access to education and healthcare is essential for advancing social justice. In doing so, society not only promotes fairness but also upholds the principles of human rights by respecting individuals' inherent dignity and entitlements.

In essence, the principles of human rights and social justice are guiding ethical frameworks that inform our responsibilities to create a more equitable and inclusive world where all individuals can lead lives of dignity, opportunity and justice.

Conclusion

In conclusion, an understanding of disability empowerment is not a luxury but a practical, social and ethical imperative. It informs the design of effective support systems, promotes inclusivity within society and upholds the principles of human rights and social justice.

This understanding lays the groundwork for empowering individuals with disabilities to lead self-determined, fulfilling lives, free from unnecessary constraints and discrimination.

2 PRINCIPLES THAT DRIVE DISABILITY EMPOWERMENT - OVERVIEW

Introduction

Disability empowerment is grounded in a set of fundamental principles that serve as the guiding force behind efforts to support and enable individuals with disabilities to lead self-determined, fulfilling lives.

These principles are not only the cornerstones of disability empowerment but also provide a framework for designing effective policies, programs and practices.

In this chapter, we will delve into the core principles that underpin disability empowerment and explore their significance in fostering a more inclusive and equitable society.

1. Individuality and Personalisation

Central to disability empowerment is the recognition of each individual's unique needs, preferences and goals.

The principle of individuality emphasises that no two individuals with disabilities are alike and their support should be tailored to their specific circumstances.

Personalisation ensures that interventions, services and support are customised to maximise an individual's potential and enhance their quality of life.

This principle challenges the one-size-fits-all approach and embraces diversity.

2. Autonomy and Informed Decision-Making

Empowerment hinges on the principle of autonomy—the right of individuals with disabilities to make choices, assert their preferences and have control over their lives.

Informed decision-making complements this principle by providing individuals and their caregivers with the information, resources and support they need to make choices about their care and support services.

It acknowledges that individuals are the experts in their own lives and should have a say in decisions that affect them.

3. Self-Determination

Self-determination is the driving force behind disability empowerment. It goes beyond autonomy by encouraging active participation in decision-making processes, including setting goals, choosing service providers and determining the level of support required.

This principle recognises that individuals with disabilities are capable of making choices that shape their lives and fosters a sense of self-direction and ownership of one's destiny.

4. Advocacy and Equal Access

Advocacy is an integral aspect of disability empowerment, advocating for the rights of individuals with disabilities and ensuring equal access to services, employment, education and opportunities.

This principle involves challenging discrimination, breaking down barriers and pushing for the development and enforcement of laws and regulations that protect these rights.

It is a powerful tool for effecting positive change on both individual and systemic levels.

5. Skill-Building and Independence

Disability empowerment recognises the importance of skill-building.

This principle involves equipping individuals with disabilities with essential life skills, such as communication, problem-solving and self-advocacy, to foster independence.

It acknowledges that skill development enhances self-confidence, self-sufficiency and the ability to actively participate in society.

6. Positive Self-Image and Pride

Promoting a positive self-image and pride is essential in disability empowerment.

This principle challenges stereotypes and misconceptions about individuals with disabilities and fosters a sense of pride and self-worth.

It recognises that a positive self-image is a critical foundation for achieving one's potential and engaging fully in society.

Conclusion

These principles collectively form the bedrock of disability empowerment, guiding efforts to create a more inclusive and equitable world for individuals with disabilities.

They emphasise the importance of recognising individuality, supporting autonomy and advocating for equal rights while nurturing self-determination, building essential skills and promoting positive self-image.

Understanding and applying these principles are essential steps toward advancing the cause of disability empowerment and creating a society where everyone can thrive.

3. INDIVIDUALITY AND PERSONALISATION

Person-Centred Care: Disability empowerment emphasises tailoring care and support services to the unique needs, preferences and goals of each individual with a disability. It shifts the focus away from a one-size-fits-all approach to care.

This approach stands in contrast to a traditional, one-size-fits-all model of care, which may not adequately address the diverse and individualised requirements of people with disabilities.

Here are some key aspects of person-centred care within the context of disability empowerment:

Individualised Care Plans:
- Person-centred care starts by conducting a thorough assessment of the individual's strengths, limitations and aspirations.
- This assessment serves as the foundation for developing a personalised care plan that addresses

their specific needs and goals.

Active Involvement:

- In this approach, individuals with disabilities are actively involved in the planning and decision-making processes related to their care.
- They have a say in setting their goals, choosing interventions and determining the level of support they require.

Respect for Autonomy:

- Person-centred care respects the autonomy and self-determination of individuals with disabilities.
- It acknowledges their right to make choices about their own lives and encourages them to express their preferences and make decisions about their care.

Flexibility:

- One of the core principles of person-centred care is flexibility.
- Care plans are designed to adapt and evolve as the individual's needs and circumstances change.
- This flexibility ensures that the care remains relevant and effective over time.

Holistic Approach:

- Rather than focusing solely on medical or physical needs, person-centred care takes a holistic approach, considering the individual's emotional, social and psychological well-being.
- It recognises that all these aspects are

interconnected and can impact a person's overall health and quality of life.

Cultural Sensitivity:

- Cultural competence and sensitivity are integral to person-centred care.
- It acknowledges and respects an individual's cultural background, values and beliefs, ensuring that care is culturally appropriate and responsive.

Communication:

- Effective communication between individuals with disabilities, their caregivers and healthcare providers is crucial.
- Person-centred care emphasises clear and open communication to ensure that everyone is on the same page and that the individual's preferences and needs are understood and met.

Empowerment:

- Empowerment is a key component of person-centred care, especially within the context of disability empowerment.
- It involves providing individuals with the tools, information and support they need to take an active role in their care and make informed decisions.

Feedback and Evaluation:

- Regular feedback from individuals with disabilities and their caregivers is essential in person-centred care
- This feedback helps evaluate the effectiveness of

care plans and make necessary adjustments to better align with the individual's evolving needs and preferences.

Quality of Life:

- Ultimately, the goal of person-centred care is to enhance the individual's quality of life.
- This approach recognises that well-being encompasses not only physical health but also emotional, social and personal fulfilment.

In summary, person-centred care in the context of disability empowerment is a holistic and individualised approach to care giving and support services.

It prioritises the dignity, autonomy and unique needs of each person with a disability, aiming to improve their overall quality of life and promote their active participation in decision-making processes related to their care.

Individuality and Personalisation in Healthcare

In the realm of healthcare, the principles of individuality and personalisation are vital in providing effective and patient-centred services.

This approach recognises that individuals with disabilities have unique healthcare needs and preferences and it emphasises the importance of tailoring care to meet those specific requirements.

Here is an overview of how individuality and

personalisation applied in healthcare for individuals with disabilities supports disability empowerment:

1. Comprehensive Assessment:

- Healthcare providers conduct comprehensive assessments of individuals with disabilities, taking into account their medical history, current health status and any disability-specific considerations.

- Individualised care plans are developed based on these assessments, addressing not only medical needs but also considering the individual's goals and preferences.

2. Communication and Decision-Making:

- Effective communication is essential. Healthcare providers ensure that individuals with disabilities are able to communicate their needs, preferences and concerns.

- Shared decision-making is encouraged, allowing individuals to actively participate in treatment decisions and choose from available options.

3. Accessibility and Accommodations:

- Healthcare facilities and equipment are designed to be accessible, accommodating individuals with various types of disabilities.

- Accommodations such as sign language interpreters, accessible examination tables and assistive technologies are readily available to ensure equitable access to healthcare services.

4. Culturally Competent Care:

- Cultural competence extends to understanding and respecting the diverse backgrounds, identities and experiences of individuals with disabilities.

- Providers are trained to provide culturally competent care that respects the unique cultural and social factors that may influence an individual's healthcare preferences and decisions.

5. Family-centred Care:

- In the case of children or individuals who require caregiver support, healthcare is often delivered in a family-centred manner.

- Families and caregivers play an active role in care decisions and their perspectives and expertise are valued.

6. Specialised Services:

- Some disabilities may require specialised healthcare services.

- Healthcare providers may collaborate with specialists, therapists and support organisations to ensure individuals receive the most appropriate and effective care.

7. Ongoing Evaluation and Adjustment:

- Healthcare plans are dynamic and subject to regular evaluation and adjustment.

- Changes are made as an individual's needs, goals or health status evolve.

8. Advocacy and Rights Protection:

- Healthcare providers often engage in advocacy efforts to ensure that individuals with disabilities have access to appropriate healthcare services and that their rights are protected.

- This may involve advocating for policy changes, supporting access to assistive devices or challenging discriminatory practices.

In summary, individuality and personalisation in healthcare for individuals with disabilities mean recognising their unique needs, preferences and goals.

It involves comprehensive assessments, accessible facilities and accommodations to ensure equitable access to care.

Effective communication, shared decision-making and culturally competent care are essential components of this approach.

By applying these principles, healthcare providers can better meet the healthcare needs of individuals with disabilities, ultimately improving their overall well-being and quality of life.

Individuality and Personalisation in Social Care

In the realm of social care, individuality and personalisation are fundamental principles that guide the provision of tailored and person-centred support for individuals with disabilities.

Recognising the uniqueness of each person and adapting care and support to their specific needs, preferences and goals is central to achieving the goals of social care.

Here is an overview of how individuality and personalisation applied in social care for individuals with disabilities supports disability empowerment:

1. Person-centred Planning:

- Person-centred planning is at the core of social care for individuals with disabilities.

- It involves collaborative discussions between the individual, their caregivers and support professionals to identify their aspirations, strengths and needs.
- The resulting care plans are highly individualised and reflect the individual's goals and priorities, taking into account their disability-related requirements.

2. Assessment and Regular Review:

- Comprehensive assessments are conducted to evaluate the individual's physical, emotional and social needs, as well as their current living arrangements and support networks.

- These assessments are regularly reviewed to ensure that the care and support provided remain aligned with the individual's evolving needs and preferences.

3. Flexibility and Adaptability:

- Social care services are designed to be flexible and adaptable.

- This means that support can be modified or adjusted to meet changing circumstances or emerging needs.

- The individual's input is actively sought when making adjustments to their care plan.

4. Empowering Choice:

- Empowering individuals to make choices about their care is a fundamental aspect of personalisation.

- Social care providers respect an individual's right to make decisions about their daily routines, activities and social interactions.

- This approach fosters a sense of ownership and control over one's life.

5. Accessible Communication:

- Effective communication is essential in personalising social care.

- Providers ensure that communication methods are accessible to individuals with disabilities, whether through assistive technologies, sign language interpreters or other means.

- Communication is tailored to the individual's preferences and needs.

6. Family and Community Involvement:

- Social care often involves family members and the broader community.

- Family-centred care recognises the importance of involving caregivers and support networks in planning and decision-making.

- Community participation is encouraged to enhance the individual's social integration and engagement.

7. Inclusive and Diverse Services:

- Social care providers offer a range of services and activities that cater to diverse interests and needs.

- These services are designed to be inclusive, ensuring that individuals with disabilities can participate fully.

- Activities are chosen based on the individual's interests and goals, promoting engagement and well-being.

8. Advocacy and Rights Protection:

- Social care providers may engage in advocacy efforts to safeguard the rights of individuals with disabilities and ensure their access to appropriate services.

- Advocacy may include addressing discrimination, securing funding or advocating for policy changes to support personalised care.

In summary, individuality and personalisation in social care for individuals with disabilities mean tailoring support to their unique needs, preferences and aspirations.

This approach involves person-centred planning, regular assessments, flexibility, empowering choice, accessible communication, family and community involvement, inclusive services and advocacy.

By adhering to these principles, social care providers can empower individuals with disabilities to lead more fulfilling and self-determined lives within their communities.

Individuality and Personalisation in Education

In the context of education, individuality and personalisation are fundamental principles that drive the design and delivery of effective and inclusive learning experiences for students with disabilities.

Recognising the uniqueness of each student and tailoring educational approaches to their specific needs, preferences and learning styles is at the heart of achieving educational goals.

Here is an overview of how individuality and personalisation applied in education for students with disabilities supports disability empowerment:

1. Individualised Education Plans (IEPs):

- Individualised Education Plans are central to providing personalised education for students with disabilities.

- These plans are developed collaboratively with input from educators, parents and, when appropriate, the students themselves.

- IEPs outline specific learning goals, accommodations and support services tailored to the individual student's needs and abilities.

2. Differentiated Instruction:

- Differentiated instruction is an instructional approach that recognises the diverse learning needs of students.

- It involves modifying teaching methods, content and assessment strategies to accommodate varying abilities and learning styles.

- Educators use differentiated instruction to ensure that each student receives instruction at a level and pace that suits them.

3. Assistive Technologies:

- The use of assistive technologies, such as screen readers, text-to-speech software or adaptive devices, plays a crucial role in personalising education for students with disabilities.

- These technologies are selected based on the individual's needs and abilities to provide access to the curriculum.

4. Accessibility and Inclusion:

- Educational environments are designed with accessibility and inclusion in mind.

- This includes physical accessibility, such as ramps and accessible classrooms, as well as digital accessibility for online learning materials.

- Inclusion promotes the integration of students with disabilities into mainstream educational settings whenever possible.

5. Individualised Support and Interventions:

- Individualised support and interventions are provided to address specific challenges or barriers that students with disabilities may encounter.

- These may include speech therapy, occupational therapy, behaviour support plans or social skills training, depending on the individual's needs.

6. Flexible Learning Pathways:

- Education for students with disabilities often involves flexible learning pathways.

- This allows students to choose courses and activities that align with their interests and goals.

- Flexibility accommodates variations in learning pace and style, empowering students to take ownership of their education.

7. Collaboration and Communication:

- Effective collaboration between educators, support staff, parents and students is essential for personalisation in education.

- Regular communication ensures that everyone is informed and engaged in supporting the student's educational journey.

8. Strength-Based Approaches:

- Personalised education emphasises a strength-based approach, recognising and building on the individual strengths and talents of each student.

- By focusing on strengths, educators and students can work together to overcome challenges and achieve educational success.

9. Advocacy and Rights Protection:

- Advocacy efforts are often needed to ensure that students with disabilities receive the educational supports and accommodations to which they are entitled.

- These efforts may involve advocating for accessible facilities, inclusive practices or the removal of barriers to learning.

In summary, individuality and personalisation in education for students with disabilities involve tailoring educational approaches to meet the unique needs, preferences and abilities of each student.

This approach encompasses individualised education plans, differentiated instruction, assistive technologies, accessibility, flexible learning pathways, collaboration, strength-based approaches and advocacy.

By embracing these principles, educators can empower students with disabilities to achieve their educational potential and thrive academically.

Individuality and Personalisation in Childcare

In the context of childcare, individuality and personalisation are foundational principles that guide the provision of nurturing and developmentally appropriate care for children with disabilities.

Recognising the unique needs, abilities and interests of each child and tailoring care and support to these specific factors are key to fostering healthy growth and development.

Here is an overview of how individuality and personalisation applied in childcare for children with disabilities supports disability empowerment:

1. Individualised Care Plans:

- Childcare providers work with parents and, when applicable, specialists to create individualised care plans for children with disabilities.

- These plans outline specific goals, accommodations and support strategies that cater to the child's unique developmental, physical and emotional needs.

2. Inclusive Environment:

- Childcare settings are designed to be inclusive, providing a welcoming and supportive atmosphere for all children.

- Inclusion promotes social interaction and learning among children with and without disabilities, fostering acceptance and understanding.

3. Adapted Activities and Materials:

- Childcare providers adapt activities, toys and learning materials to ensure that children with disabilities can actively participate.

- Modifications may include providing sensory-friendly materials, offering assistive devices or adjusting the environment for mobility and accessibility.

4. Communication and Collaboration:

- Effective communication and collaboration between childcare providers, parents, therapists and specialists are fundamental to personalisation.

- Regular updates and feedback ensure that the child's

care and developmental progress are well-coordinated and tailored to their evolving needs.

5. Individualised Learning Support:

- Childcare providers offer individualised learning support to help children with disabilities reach their developmental milestones.

- This may involve speech therapy, physical therapy, occupational therapy or specialised teaching methods based on the child's strengths and challenges.

6. Encouraging Self-Expression:

- Personalisation encourages children to express themselves in ways that suit their abilities, be it through communication devices, gestures or alternative forms of expression.

- The goal is to nurture each child's unique voice and personality.

7. Inclusive Play and Socialisation:

- Childcare settings prioritise inclusive play and socialisation opportunities.

- Play-based activities and group interactions help children with disabilities build social skills, self-confidence and a sense of belonging.

8. Supportive Transitions:

- Childcare providers assist children with disabilities in transitioning to new developmental stages or educational settings.

- This includes preparing children for kindergarten or school and ensuring that support services continue seamlessly.

9. Advocacy and Rights Protection:

- Advocacy efforts are often needed to ensure that children with disabilities receive the appropriate care and educational support.

- Childcare providers may advocate for accessible facilities, trained staff and policies that promote inclusivity.

In summary, individuality and personalisation in childcare for children with disabilities involve creating an environment where each child's unique needs and strengths are recognised and supported.

This approach includes individualised care plans, inclusive environments, adapted activities, effective communication, individualised learning support, self-expression encouragement, inclusive play and advocacy.

By embracing these principles, childcare providers can help children with disabilities thrive, grow and develop to their fullest potential.

4 AUTONOMY AND INFORMED DECISION MAKING

Autonomy

Autonomy refers to the ability and right of individuals to make independent decisions and have control over their own lives. It's a fundamental principle in various domains, including healthcare, social services, education and personal relationships.

Autonomy recognises that individuals have unique needs, preferences and values and it empowers them to make choices that align with these aspects of their identity.

Here's what autonomy entails:

Informed Decision-Making:

- Autonomy involves making choices based on comprehensive and accurate information.

- Individuals have the right to receive clear and accessible information about available options, potential risks and benefits, allowing them to make informed decisions.

Respect for Preferences:

- Autonomy respects an individual's preferences and values, even if they differ from what others might choose.

- It recognises that there is no one-size-fits-all approach to decision-making.

Freedom of Choice:

- Autonomy provides individuals with the freedom to choose among various options, whether they pertain to their healthcare, lifestyle, education or other aspects of life.

- It extends to choices related to personal relationships and daily activities.

Consent:

- In healthcare and various service settings, autonomy often involves obtaining informed consent from individuals before providing a particular treatment, intervention or service.

- Consent ensures that individuals actively agree to what happens to them.

Support for Decision-Making:

- Some individuals may require support to exercise their autonomy fully.

- This support can come from family members, friends, advocates or professionals trained in supported decision-making.

- The goal is to ensure that individuals are still the ultimate decision-makers.

Privacy and Confidentiality:

- Autonomy encompasses the right to privacy and confidentiality.

- Individuals should have control over their personal information and who has access to it.

Advocacy for Rights:

- Autonomy often involves advocating for and protecting an individual's rights, particularly when those rights are at risk of being violated or when external factors threaten an individual's decision-making capacity.

Continuous Review:

- Autonomy isn't static; it evolves as circumstances change.

- Periodic reviews of decisions and choices may be necessary to ensure that they remain aligned with an individual's current preferences and needs.

Empowerment:

- Autonomy empowers individuals to take an active role in their lives.

- It fosters independence and self-determination, promoting a sense of control over one's destiny.

Legal Protections:

- Laws and regulations exist to protect an individual's autonomy, especially in situations where they may be vulnerable or at risk of exploitation.

Person-centred Approaches:

- Person-centred care and services emphasise autonomy by tailoring support to the unique needs, preferences and goals of each individual.

- This approach ensures that the person remains at the centre of decision-making.

In summary, autonomy is a core principle that recognises and respects an individual's right to make choices and decisions that affect their life.

It's about providing information, support and a safe space for individuals to assert their preferences, values and desires, ultimately enabling them to lead a more self-directed and fulfilling life.

Informed Decision-Making

Informed decision-making is a critical component of person-centred care and disability empowerment.

It entails providing individuals with disabilities, as well as their families or caregivers when applicable, with the necessary information and resources to make informed choices about their care and support services.

Here's a closer look at what this entails:

Access to Information:

- Individuals with disabilities have the right to access clear and understandable information about their health, care options and available services.

- This information should be provided in accessible formats, taking into consideration any communication or accessibility needs of the individual.

Educational Support:

- Education is a key aspect of informed decision-making.

- Individuals should be offered educational resources and opportunities to learn about their conditions, treatment options and potential outcomes.

- This can include written materials, verbal explanations, videos or online resources.

Exploration of Options:

- Informed decision-making involves exploring a range of options and alternatives for care and support services. Individuals should be presented with choices that align with their goals and preferences, allowing them to make decisions that suit their unique needs.

Understanding Risks and Benefits:

- Individuals should be informed about the potential risks and benefits associated with different care and treatment options.

- This includes discussing potential side effects, complications and expected outcomes.

- This information allows individuals to weigh the pros and cons of each choice.

Clarification of Goals and Values:

- The decision-making process should involve discussions about an individual's personal values, beliefs and long-term goals.

- This helps align care plans with the individual's

broader aspirations and desires for their life.

Informed Consent:

- In healthcare settings, informed consent is a legal and ethical requirement.
- It means that individuals must fully understand the proposed treatments or interventions, their alternatives and potential risks before agreeing to them.
- Informed consent ensures that individuals actively participate in their care decisions.

Shared Decision-Making:

- Shared decision-making is a collaborative approach in which individuals, their families or caregivers and healthcare professionals work together to make decisions.
- It recognises that individuals are experts in their own lives and values their input in the decision-making process.

Ongoing Communication:

- Informed decision-making is not a one-time event but an ongoing process. Individuals should have the opportunity to revisit and revise their decisions as their circumstances, preferences and needs change over time.

Advocacy and Support:

- Individuals may require advocacy and support to navigate complex healthcare systems and understand their options fully.

- Advocates or support professionals can help individuals with disabilities and their families navigate the decision-making process.

Respect for Choices:

- Ultimately, informed decision-making respects an individual's right to make choices that align with their values and preferences, even if those choices differ from what others might consider the "best" option.
- It recognises and respects the autonomy of the individual.

In summary, informed decision-making is a core principle of person-centred care and disability empowerment.

It ensures that individuals with disabilities are active participants in decisions related to their care and support and it promotes their autonomy and well-being by providing them with the information and resources they need to make choices that reflect their individual goals and preferences.

Autonomy and Informed Decision-Making in Healthcare

In healthcare, autonomy and informed decision-making are fundamental principles that empower individuals to actively participate in their own care and treatment decisions.

These principles uphold an individual's right to make choices about their healthcare based on accurate information and personal preferences.

Here is an overview of how autonomy and informed decision-making applied in healthcare promotes disability empowerment:

1. Respect for Autonomy:

- Autonomy refers to an individual's right to make decisions about their own life, including healthcare choices.

- Healthcare providers and professionals respect this autonomy by recognising the patient as the ultimate decision-maker regarding their treatment.

- Regardless of a patient's disability, healthcare providers prioritise their right to express preferences and make choices related to their health.

2. Informed Consent:

- Informed consent is a key component of autonomy and informed decision-making.

- Before any medical procedure or treatment, healthcare providers ensure that patients (or their legal guardians) fully understand the potential benefits, risks and alternatives.

- For individuals with disabilities, healthcare providers take extra steps to facilitate comprehension, which may involve using plain language, visual aids or communication supports.

3. Shared Decision-Making:

- Shared decision-making is a collaborative approach in which healthcare providers and patients (and often their families or caregivers) work together to make healthcare decisions.

- It acknowledges that individuals with disabilities and their support networks possess valuable insights and preferences that inform the decision-making process.

4. Accessible Information:

- Accessibility is crucial in ensuring that individuals with disabilities have the information they need to make informed decisions.

- Healthcare providers provide information in accessible formats, such as Braille, large print, easy-to-read materials or through assistive technologies.

5. Effective Communication:

- Effective communication is essential to enable individuals with disabilities to express their preferences and concerns.

- Healthcare providers use communication methods and tools that align with the individual's abilities, such as sign language interpreters or communication boards.

6. Patient Education:

- Healthcare providers engage in patient education to empower individuals with disabilities with the knowledge necessary to make informed decisions.

- This education covers their condition, treatment options, potential side effects and long-term implications.

7. Support for Decision-Making:

- Some individuals with disabilities may require additional support to make healthcare decisions.

- In such cases, healthcare providers involve family members, caregivers or patient advocates to ensure the individual's preferences are respected.

8. Continual Reassessment:

- Autonomy and informed decision-making are not static; they evolve with changes in a person's health and life circumstances.
- Healthcare providers continually reassess the individual's capacity to make decisions and adjust their approach accordingly.

9. Legal Protections:

- Legal protections, such as healthcare proxies and advance directives, are used when individuals are unable to make decisions due to their disability or health condition.

- These legal instruments allow individuals to appoint someone they trust to make healthcare decisions on their behalf.

In summary, autonomy and informed decision-making in healthcare are principles that emphasise an individual's right to be involved in decisions about their health and treatment.

This approach respects their preferences, facilitates understanding and ensures that healthcare information is accessible and communicated effectively.

By upholding these principles, healthcare providers enable individuals with disabilities to take an active role in their healthcare journey, promoting their overall well-being and quality of life.

Autonomy and Informed Decision-Making in Social Care

In the field of social care, autonomy and informed decision-making are foundational principles that empower individuals with disabilities to actively shape their own care plans and support services.

These principles uphold an individual's right to make choices about their social care based on accurate information and personal preferences.

Here is an overview of how autonomy and informed decision-making applied in social care promotes disability empowerment:

1. Person-centred Planning:

- Person-centred planning is at the core of social care for individuals with disabilities.

- It involves collaborative discussions between the individual, their caregivers and support professionals to identify their aspirations, strengths and needs.

- The resulting care plans are highly individualised and reflect the individual's goals and priorities, taking into account their disability-related requirements.

2. Informed Choice:

- Empowering individuals with disabilities to make informed choices about their social care is a key aspect of autonomy.

- It entails providing clear and accessible information about available support services, benefits and alternatives.

- Individuals are encouraged to explore their options and express their preferences.

3. Accessibility of Information:

- Ensuring that information is accessible is crucial for informed decision-making.

- Social care providers present information in formats that individuals with disabilities can understand and use.

- This may include using plain language, providing information in multiple formats (e.g., large print, Braille, easy-to-read materials) or utilising assistive technologies.

4. Effective Communication:

- Effective communication is essential to enable individuals with disabilities to express their preferences, concerns and questions.

- Social care providers use communication methods that align with the individual's abilities, including sign language interpreters, communication boards or augmentative and alternative communication (AAC) devices.

5. Support for Decision-Making:

- Recognising that some individuals with disabilities may require support to make decisions, social care providers offer assistance.

- This support may come from family members, friends, advocates or professionals trained in supported decision-making.

6. Regular Review and Reassessment:

- Autonomy and informed decision-making are dynamic processes.

- Social care plans are reviewed and reassessed regularly to ensure that they remain aligned with the individual's evolving needs, goals and preferences.

- Adjustments are made as necessary to accommodate changes in circumstances.

7. Advocacy for Rights Protection:

- Social care providers may engage in advocacy efforts to protect the rights of individuals with disabilities and ensure they have access to the support services and accommodations they require.

- Advocacy can involve challenging discriminatory practices or advocating for policy changes.

8. Independence and Empowerment:

- Autonomy in social care aims to foster independence and empowerment.

- It recognises that individuals with disabilities have

the ability to make meaningful choices that impact their lives.

- Support is provided to help individuals build skills and confidence to exercise their autonomy effectively.

9. Person-centred Outcomes:

- Social care outcomes are based on the individual's goals and preferences.

- Success is measured by the extent to which the individual's choices and aspirations are realised.

- This approach shifts the focus from standardised outcomes to outcomes that are personally meaningful to the individual.

In summary, autonomy and informed decision-making in social care for individuals with disabilities mean respecting their right to actively participate in shaping their own support services and care plans.

This approach involves person-centred planning, informed choice, accessibility of information, effective communication, support for decision-making, regular review, advocacy, independence and person-centred outcomes.

By upholding these principles, social care providers empower individuals with disabilities to lead self-determined, fulfilling lives within their communities.

Autonomy and Informed Decision-Making in Education

In the realm of education, autonomy and informed decision-making are fundamental principles that empower students with disabilities to actively participate in shaping their own learning experiences.

These principles recognise the right of students to make choices about their education based on accurate information and personal preferences.

Here is an overview of how autonomy and informed decision-making applied in education for students with disabilities promotes disability empowerment:

1. Individualised Education Plans (IEPs):

- Individualised Education Plans (IEPs) are central to providing students with disabilities the autonomy to tailor their educational journey.
- These plans are collaboratively developed with input from educators, parents and, when applicable, the students themselves.

- IEPs outline specific learning goals, accommodations and support services tailored to the individual student's needs and abilities.

2. Student-centred Learning:

- Autonomy in education encourages student-centred learning, where students actively engage in decision-making about their education.

- This approach allows students to choose topics of interest, learning methods and even the pace at which they progress through curriculum content.

3. Accessible Information:

- Accessibility is crucial to informed decision-making in education.

- Schools provide information about educational options, resources and programs in formats that students with disabilities can understand and use.

- Materials are made accessible through means such as Braille, large print, accessible websites or assistive technologies.

4. Effective Communication:

- Effective communication ensures that students with disabilities can express their preferences and concerns regarding their education.

- Schools use communication methods and tools that align with the student's abilities, including sign language interpreters, communication boards or augmentative and alternative communication (AAC) devices.

5. Support for Decision-Making:

- Recognising that some students with disabilities may require support to make educational decisions, schools offer assistance.

- This support may come from teachers, counsellors or educational advocates who work collaboratively with the student.

6. Regular Student Involvement:

- Autonomy and informed decision-making involve

regular involvement of the student in their educational planning and goal-setting.

- As students grow and their needs change, their preferences and goals are continually taken into account and adjusted accordingly.

7. Advocacy for Rights Protection:

- Educational institutions often engage in advocacy efforts to protect the rights of students with disabilities and ensure they have access to appropriate educational services and accommodations.

- Advocacy may include addressing discrimination, securing funding or advocating for policy changes that promote inclusive education.

8. Inclusive and Diverse Learning Environments:

- Autonomy and informed decision-making support the creation of inclusive and diverse learning environments.

- Students with disabilities are encouraged to actively participate in inclusive classrooms where their unique abilities and perspectives are valued.

9. Student-Led Initiatives:

- Encouraging students to take the lead in initiatives related to their education is an essential aspect of autonomy.

- This may include involvement in extracurricular activities, advocacy groups or decision-making committees.

In summary, autonomy and informed decision-making in education for students with disabilities mean recognising their right to actively participate in decisions about their learning experiences.

This approach involves individualised education plans, student-centred learning, accessible information, effective communication, support for decision-making, regular student involvement, advocacy, inclusive environments and student-led initiatives.

By upholding these principles, educational institutions empower students with disabilities to take ownership of their education, achieve their academic goals and thrive as independent learners.

Autonomy and Informed Decision-Making in Childcare

In the context of childcare, autonomy and informed decision-making are essential principles that promote the well-being and development of children with disabilities.

These principles recognise the right of children and their families to actively shape their own childcare experiences based on accurate information and personal preferences.

Here is an overview of how autonomy and informed decision-making applied in childcare for children with disabilities promotes disability empowerment:

1. Family-centred Approach:

- A family-centred approach in childcare recognises that parents and caregivers play a crucial role in decision-making for children with disabilities.

- It involves collaborative discussions between families, childcare providers and specialists to create a care plan that aligns with the child's unique needs and family preferences.

2. Individualised Care Plans:

- Childcare providers work with parents and specialists to develop individualised care plans for children with disabilities.

- These plans outline specific goals, accommodations and support strategies that cater to the child's unique developmental, physical and emotional needs.

3. Inclusive Environments:

- Childcare settings are designed to be inclusive, providing a welcoming and supportive atmosphere for all children.

- Inclusion promotes social interaction and learning among children with and without disabilities, fostering acceptance and understanding.

4. Accessible Information:

- Ensuring that information is accessible is vital for informed decision-making in childcare.

- Childcare providers provide information about care options, developmental resources and programs in formats that parents and caregivers can understand and use.

- Materials are made accessible through means such as plain language, visual aids or digital accessibility features.

5. Effective Communication:

- Effective communication ensures that parents, caregivers and children with disabilities can express their preferences, concerns and questions.

- Childcare providers use communication methods that align with the child's abilities, including sign language, communication boards or augmentative and alternative communication (AAC) devices.

6. Support for Decision-Making:

- Recognising that parents and caregivers may require support to make decisions for children with disabilities, childcare providers offer assistance.

- This support may include guidance from childcare specialists, therapists or advocacy organisations.

7. Individualised Learning and Play:

- Autonomy in childcare promotes individualised learning and play experiences for children with disabilities.

- Childcare providers tailor activities, toys and learning materials to cater to the child's specific abilities and interests.

8. Advocacy for Rights Protection:

- Childcare providers may engage in advocacy efforts to protect the rights of children with disabilities and ensure they have access to appropriate childcare services and accommodations.

- Advocacy may involve addressing discrimination, securing funding or advocating for policy changes to promote inclusive childcare.

9. Transition Support:

- Childcare providers assist children with disabilities in transitioning to new developmental stages or educational settings.

- This includes preparing children for school or other childcare settings and ensuring that support services continue seamlessly.

In summary, autonomy and informed decision-making in childcare for children with disabilities mean recognising the rights of families and children to actively participate in decisions about their childcare experiences.

This approach involves family-centred care, individualised care plans, inclusive environments, accessible information, effective communication, support for decision-making, individualised learning and play, advocacy and transition support.

By upholding these principles, childcare providers empower families and children with disabilities to access quality care and support that promotes their overall well-being and development.

5 SELF-DETERMINATION

Self-Determination

Self-determination is a crucial aspect of empowerment, especially within the context of disability services and care.

It refers to the ability and right of individuals to make choices and decisions about their own lives, including decisions related to their care plans.

Here's a deeper look at self-determination:

Autonomy:

- Self-determination places a strong emphasis on autonomy, which means that individuals have the authority to make decisions about their own lives and exercise control over their choices.

- This includes decisions about daily routines, living arrangements and the services they receive.

Setting Personal Goals:

- Self-determination encourages individuals to identify and set their own personal goals.
- These goals can encompass various aspects of life, including health, education, employment, social relationships and more.
- The process of setting goals empowers individuals to define what they want to achieve.

Choice in Service Providers:

- Individuals should have the freedom to choose their service providers.
- This allows them to select professionals and caregivers they feel comfortable with and who align with their values and needs.
- It also fosters a sense of control over their support network.

Individualised Care Plans:

- Self-determination involves the development of individualised care plans that are tailored to the specific goals and preferences of the person with a disability.
- These plans should be flexible and responsive to changing needs and circumstances.

Active Participation:

- Individuals are encouraged and supported in actively participating in decision-making processes related to their care.

- This participation can range from choosing meal preferences to determining the level of assistance needed with daily activities.

Informed Choices:

- To exercise self-determination effectively, individuals need access to information about available options, risks and benefits.
- This information enables them to make informed choices that align with their values and aspirations.

Self-Advocacy:

- Self-determination often goes hand in hand with self-advocacy.
- Individuals are empowered to speak up for their needs and preferences, express concerns and assert their rights.
- This may involve seeking assistance from advocacy organisations or support professionals.

Support for Decision-Making:

- While self-determination emphasises independence, it also recognises that some individuals may require support to make decisions.
- This support should be provided in a way that respects the individual's autonomy and preferences.

Legal and Ethical Framework:

- Self-determination is supported by legal and ethical principles that uphold the rights of individuals with disabilities to have control over their lives and make choices in their best interest.

Quality of Life:

- Ultimately, self-determination is about enhancing an individual's quality of life.
- It allows individuals to pursue their own interests, engage in activities they enjoy and lead fulfilling lives on their own terms.

In summary, self-determination is a central element of empowerment for individuals with disabilities.

It recognises their capacity to make choices, set goals and actively participate in decision-making processes regarding their care and support services.

By promoting self-determination, caregivers, service providers and society at large can better enable individuals with disabilities to lead self-directed, meaningful lives.

Self-Determination in Healthcare

In the realm of healthcare, self-determination is a critical principle that recognises the autonomy and agency of individuals with disabilities in making decisions about their own medical care and well-being.

Self-determination goes beyond informed consent; it emphasises the active involvement of individuals with disabilities in every aspect of their healthcare journey.

Here is an overview of how self-determination applied in healthcare for individuals with disabilities promotes disability empowerment:

1. Decision-Making Partnerships:

- Self-determination in healthcare promotes collaborative decision-making partnerships between healthcare providers and individuals with disabilities.

- It involves open and respectful communication where individuals are encouraged to express their preferences, concerns and goals.

2. Involvement in Care Planning:

- Individuals with disabilities actively participate in the development of their care plans.

- They work alongside healthcare providers to set health goals, choose treatment options and discuss the approach to care that best suits their needs.

3. Informed Choice:

- Self-determination hinges on informed choice. Individuals with disabilities receive comprehensive information about their medical conditions, treatment options, potential risks and benefits.

- This information is presented in accessible formats that align with the individual's abilities.

4. Support for Decision-Making:

- Recognising that some individuals with disabilities may require support to make healthcare decisions, healthcare providers ensure that assistance is available.

- Support can come from family members, friends or

healthcare advocates who work alongside the individual to facilitate informed choices.

5. Communication Accessibility:

- Effective communication is key to self-determination.

- Healthcare providers employ communication methods and tools that cater to the individual's abilities, including sign language interpreters, communication boards or assistive communication devices.

6. Advance Directives:

- Advance directives allow individuals to document their healthcare preferences in advance, especially regarding end-of-life decisions.

- This legal instrument ensures that their wishes are respected even when they may be unable to communicate them later.

7. Continuity of Care:

- Self-determination also extends to decisions about continuity of care and treatment.

- Individuals with disabilities have the right to choose their healthcare providers and to be informed about any changes in their care plan.

8. Advocacy for Rights Protection:

- Healthcare providers and advocates may engage in advocacy efforts to safeguard the rights of individuals with disabilities.

- This advocacy can involve addressing discrimination, advocating for accessible healthcare facilities or challenging policies that hinder self-determination.

9. Promoting Health Literacy:

- Self-determination in healthcare includes efforts to promote health literacy among individuals with disabilities.

- Education and resources are provided to help them understand their health conditions and make informed decisions.

In summary, self-determination in healthcare is a principle that empowers individuals with disabilities to actively participate in their healthcare decisions.

This approach involves decision-making partnerships, involvement in care planning, informed choice, support for decision-making, communication accessibility, advance directives, continuity of care, advocacy and health literacy promotion.

By upholding these principles, healthcare providers enable individuals with disabilities to exercise control over their healthcare, make choices aligned with their values and preferences and ultimately enhance their overall well-being and quality of life.

Self-Determination in Social Care

In the field of social care, self-determination is a foundational principle that empowers individuals with disabilities to actively shape their own care plans and support services.

It acknowledges their right to make decisions about their social care based on their personal preferences and goals.

Here is an overview of how self-determination applied in social care promotes disability empowerment:

1. Person-centred Planning:

- Person-centred planning is central to self-determination in social care.

- It involves collaborative discussions between individuals with disabilities, their caregivers and support professionals to identify their aspirations, strengths and needs.

- The resulting care plans are highly individualised and reflect the individual's goals and priorities.

2. Informed Choice:

- Self-determination in social care encourages individuals with disabilities to make informed choices about their care and support services.

- Information about available support options, benefits and alternatives is provided in accessible formats, ensuring that individuals can explore and express their preferences.

3. Support for Decision-Making:

- Recognising that some individuals with disabilities may require support to make decisions, social care providers offer assistance.

- Support may come from family members, friends or advocates who work collaboratively with the individual to ensure their choices are respected.

4. Effective Communication:

- Effective communication is fundamental to self-determination.

- Social care providers use communication methods and tools that align with the individual's abilities, including sign language, communication boards or assistive communication devices.

5. Advocacy for Rights Protection:

- Social care providers may engage in advocacy efforts to protect the rights of individuals with disabilities and ensure they have access to appropriate social care services and accommodations.

- Advocacy can involve addressing discrimination, securing funding or advocating for policy changes that promote inclusive social care.

6. Continual Reassessment:

- Self-determination is a dynamic process in social care.

- Care plans are reviewed and reassessed regularly to ensure that they remain aligned with the individual's evolving needs, goals and preferences.

- Adjustments are made as necessary to accommodate changes in circumstances.

7. Independence and Empowerment:

- Self-determination aims to foster independence and empowerment.

- It recognises that individuals with disabilities have the ability to make meaningful choices that impact their lives.

- Support is provided to help individuals build skills and confidence to exercise their self-determination effectively.

8. Inclusive and Diverse Support:

- Self-determination promotes the creation of inclusive and diverse support networks.

- Individuals with disabilities are encouraged to actively participate in their communities, accessing support services that align with their unique abilities and goals.

9. Person-centred Outcomes:

- Social care outcomes are based on the individual's goals and preferences.

- Success is measured by the extent to which the individual's choices and aspirations are realised.

- This approach shifts the focus from standardised outcomes to outcomes that are personally meaningful to the individual.

In summary, self-determination in social care is a principle that recognises the rights of individuals with disabilities to actively participate in decisions about their care plans and support services.

This approach involves person-centred planning, informed choice, support for decision-making, effective communication, advocacy, continual reassessment, independence, inclusive support and person-centred outcomes.

By upholding these principles, social care providers empower individuals with disabilities to lead self-determined, fulfilling lives within their communities.

Self-Determination in Education

In the realm of education, self-determination is a fundamental principle that recognises the autonomy and agency of students with disabilities in making choices about their own learning experiences and educational goals.

This principle goes beyond merely accommodating students; it empowers them to actively participate in shaping their educational journey.

Here is an overview of how self-determination applied in education for students with disabilities promotes disability empowerment:

1. Student-centred Learning:

- Self-determination in education promotes student-centred learning, where students with disabilities have the opportunity to take an active role in their educational experiences.

- It allows students to voice their preferences, interests and goals, leading to more engaging and personalised learning.

2. Individualised Education Plans (IEPs):

- Individualised Education Plans (IEPs) are a cornerstone of self-determination in education.

- These plans are collaboratively developed with input from students, parents, educators and, when applicable, specialists.

- IEPs outline specific learning goals, accommodations and support services tailored to the student's unique needs and abilities.

3. Informed Decision-Making:

- Students with disabilities are encouraged to engage in informed decision-making about their education.
- This includes decisions about coursework, extracurricular activities and goals beyond the classroom.

- Schools provide information in accessible formats to ensure that students can make choices based on accurate information.

4. Support for Decision-Making:

- Recognising that some students with disabilities may require support to make educational decisions, schools offer assistance.

- This support may come from teachers, counsellors or educational advocates who work collaboratively with the student to facilitate informed choices.

5. Communication Accessibility:

- Effective communication is paramount to self-determination in education.

- Schools employ communication methods and tools that cater to the student's abilities, including sign language interpreters, communication boards or assistive communication devices.

6. Transition Planning:

- Self-determination extends to decisions about transitions, such as moving from one educational level to another or transitioning to post-school life.

- Transition planning involves preparing students for these changes and ensuring that their preferences and goals are considered.

7. Advocacy and Self-Advocacy:

- Schools encourage students with disabilities to become advocates for themselves.

- Self-advocacy skills empower students to communicate their needs, seek accommodations and assert their rights.

- Additionally, schools may engage in advocacy efforts to protect the rights of students with disabilities and ensure they have access to inclusive education.

8. Inclusive and Diverse Learning Environments:

- Self-determination promotes the creation of inclusive and diverse learning environments.

- Students with disabilities are encouraged to actively participate in inclusive classrooms where their unique abilities and perspectives are valued.

9. Measuring Success by Personal Goals:

- The success of self-determination in education is measured by the extent to which students' personal goals and aspirations are achieved.

- This approach shifts the focus from standardised outcomes to outcomes that are personally meaningful to the student.

In summary, self-determination in education is a principle that empowers students with disabilities to take an active role in their educational journey.

This approach involves student-centred learning, individualised education plans, informed decision-making, support for decision-making, communication accessibility, transition planning, advocacy and self-advocacy, inclusive environments and personal goal achievement.

By upholding these principles, educational institutions enable students with disabilities to take ownership of their education, achieve their academic goals and develop into self-determined learners who can advocate for their needs and preferences.

Self-Determination in Childcare

In the context of childcare, self-determination is a foundational principle that recognises the autonomy and agency of children with disabilities and their families in making decisions about their childcare experiences and support services.

This principle promotes an environment where children's

voices are valued and their preferences and goals are taken into account.

Here is an overview of how self-determination applied in childcare for children with disabilities promotes disability empowerment:

1. Family-centred Approach:

- A family-centred approach in childcare recognises that parents and caregivers play a crucial role in decision-making for children with disabilities.

- It involves collaborative discussions between families, childcare providers and specialists to create a childcare plan that aligns with the child's unique needs and family preferences.

2. Individualised Care Plans:

- Childcare providers work with parents and specialists to develop individualised care plans for children with disabilities.

- These plans outline specific goals, accommodations and support strategies that cater to the child's unique developmental, physical and emotional needs.

3. Inclusive Environments:

- Childcare settings are designed to be inclusive, providing a welcoming and supportive atmosphere for all children.

- Inclusion promotes social interaction and learning among children with and without disabilities, fostering acceptance and understanding.

4. Encouraging Children's Voices:

- Self-determination in childcare encourages children with disabilities to have a say in their childcare experiences.

- It recognises that even young children can express preferences and choices.

- Childcare providers create opportunities for children to make decisions about activities, playtime and routines.

5. Communication Accessibility:

- Effective communication is vital to self-determination. Childcare providers employ communication methods and tools that cater to the child's abilities, including sign language, communication boards or assistive communication devices.

6. Support for Decision-Making:

- Recognising that some children with disabilities may require support to make decisions, childcare providers offer assistance.

- Support may come from family members, friends or childcare specialists who work alongside the child to facilitate choices.

7. Advocacy for Rights Protection:

- Childcare providers may engage in advocacy efforts to protect the rights of children with disabilities and ensure they have access to appropriate childcare services and accommodations.

- Advocacy may include addressing discrimination, securing funding or advocating for policy changes that promote inclusive childcare.

8. Independence and Empowerment:

- Self-determination aims to foster independence and empowerment. It recognises that children with disabilities have the ability to make meaningful choices that impact their experiences.

- Support is provided to help children build confidence and self-advocacy skills.

9. Transition Support:

- Childcare providers assist children with disabilities in transitioning to new developmental stages or educational settings.

- This includes preparing children for school or other childcare settings and ensuring that support services continue seamlessly.

In summary, self-determination in childcare is a principle that empowers children with disabilities and their families to actively participate in decisions about their childcare experiences.

This approach involves a family-centred approach, individualised care plans, inclusive environments, encouraging children's voices, communication accessibility, support for decision-making, advocacy, independence and empowerment and transition support.

By upholding these principles, childcare providers empower families and children with disabilities to access quality care and support that promotes their overall well-being and development.

6 ADVOCACY

Advocacy

Advocacy plays a vital role in disability empowerment by promoting the rights, inclusion and equal opportunities of people with disabilities. Advocates and advocacy organisations work to raise awareness, challenge discriminatory practices and influence policy changes.

Here are key aspects of advocacy within the context of disability empowerment:

Rights Protection:

- Advocacy efforts focus on protecting and promoting the rights of individuals with disabilities.
- These rights may include civil rights, healthcare access, education, employment, housing and more.
- Advocates work to ensure that these rights are upheld and respected.

Equal Access:

- Advocacy strives to eliminate barriers that prevent individuals with disabilities from accessing essential services, opportunities and resources.
- This includes advocating for accessible public transportation, buildings, websites and communication methods.

Inclusive Education:

- Advocates promote inclusive education practices that allow students with disabilities to be educated alongside their non-disabled peers.
- They challenge segregated schooling and push for accommodations that support learning needs.

Employment Opportunities:

- Advocacy efforts aim to create a more inclusive workforce by advocating for equal employment opportunities and reasonable accommodations for individuals with disabilities.
- This includes challenging workplace discrimination and promoting diversity and inclusion.

Healthcare Access:

- Advocates work to ensure that individuals with disabilities have equal access to healthcare services, including preventive care, medical treatment and rehabilitation services.
- They may also advocate for improvements in healthcare facilities' accessibility.

Legal Protections:

- Advocacy often involves pushing for the development and enforcement of laws and regulations that protect the rights of people with disabilities.
- This includes laws like the Equality Act, The Special Educational Needs and Disability (SEND) Code of Practice, Access to Work Scheme

Policy Change:

- Advocates may engage in lobbying efforts and work with policymakers to influence legislation and policies that impact individuals with disabilities.
- They aim to create a legal framework that supports empowerment and inclusion.

Community Integration:

- Advocacy encourages the integration of individuals with disabilities into their communities.
- This includes promoting community-based living arrangements over institutionalisation and fostering social inclusion.

Awareness and Education:

- Advocates raise awareness about the challenges faced by people with disabilities and the importance of disability rights.
- They conduct educational campaigns to dispel myths and misconceptions about disabilities.

Challenging Discrimination:

- Advocacy organisations often take legal action to challenge discrimination and human rights violations against people with disabilities.

- They may provide legal support to individuals facing discrimination.

Self-Advocacy:

- Empowering individuals with disabilities to become self-advocates is an essential aspect of advocacy.
- This involves teaching individuals how to assert their rights, communicate their needs and advocate for themselves.

Coalition Building:

- Advocacy groups often collaborate with other organisations and communities to build a broader movement for disability rights.
- This collective action can have a more significant impact on policy change and social attitudes.

Advocacy efforts are essential in the pursuit of disability empowerment because they aim to create a more inclusive and equitable society where individuals with disabilities can participate fully in all aspects of life.

By advocating for change at various levels—individual, community, institutional and legislative—advocates contribute to breaking down barriers and advancing the rights and well-being of people with disabilities.

Advocacy and Equal Access in Healthcare

Advocacy and equal access are critical components of healthcare, ensuring that individuals, including those with disabilities, receive fair and equitable treatment and have their rights protected. In healthcare, advocacy involves promoting the interests, rights and well-being of patients, especially those who may face barriers to accessing quality care.

Here is an overview of advocacy and equal access in healthcare, particularly for individuals with disabilities:

1. Addressing Healthcare Disparities:

- Advocacy in healthcare aims to address healthcare disparities that individuals with disabilities may experience.

- These disparities can include difficulties in accessing healthcare services, receiving appropriate accommodations or encountering discriminatory attitudes.

2. Legal Protections:

- Legal frameworks protect the rights of individuals with disabilities in healthcare settings.

- Advocates work to ensure that healthcare facilities and providers comply with these laws, providing accessible environments and services.

3. Accessible Facilities and Equipment:

- Advocacy efforts focus on making healthcare facilities and equipment accessible to individuals with disabilities.

- This includes ensuring that medical offices, hospitals and clinics have ramps, accessible exam tables and other accommodations.

4. Communication Accessibility:

- Advocacy includes advocating for effective communication between healthcare providers and patients with disabilities.

- This may involve providing sign language interpreters, communication boards or assistive communication devices.

5. Informed Consent and Decision-Making:

- Advocacy emphasises the importance of informed consent, ensuring that individuals with disabilities have access to information about their medical conditions, treatment options and potential risks and benefits.

- Supported decision-making may be facilitated for those who require assistance in making healthcare choices.

6. Access to Specialised Care:

- Advocates work to ensure that individuals with disabilities have equal access to specialised care and services tailored to their unique needs, whether they pertain to physical, developmental or mental health conditions.

7. Protection from Discrimination:

- Advocacy efforts focus on protecting individuals with disabilities from discrimination in healthcare settings.

- This includes challenging discriminatory practices and attitudes that may result in subpar care or unequal treatment.

8. Promoting Inclusive Healthcare Practices:

- Advocacy promotes the adoption of inclusive healthcare practices, where healthcare providers receive training on how to provide respectful and culturally sensitive care to individuals with disabilities.

9. Support in Navigating the Healthcare System:

- Advocates often provide support to individuals with disabilities in navigating the complex healthcare system.

- This may involve helping with insurance claims, appointment scheduling and understanding medical information.

10. Raising Awareness:

- Advocacy raises awareness about the healthcare needs and challenges faced by individuals with disabilities.

- This includes educating healthcare providers and the public about disability-related issues.

11. Ensuring Accommodations:

- Advocates ensure that individuals with disabilities receive the necessary accommodations to fully participate in healthcare decisions, treatments and therapies.

12. Policy Change and Reform:

- Advocacy often extends to advocating for policy changes and reforms that enhance access to healthcare services, improve care quality and protect the rights of individuals with disabilities.

In summary, advocacy and equal access in healthcare for individuals with disabilities are essential for ensuring that they receive the same quality of care as anyone else.

These efforts encompass addressing disparities, ensuring legal protections, promoting accessibility, facilitating communication, supporting informed decision-making, combating discrimination and raising awareness.

Through advocacy and equal access initiatives, individuals with disabilities can access healthcare services that align with their unique needs and promote their overall well-being.

Advocacy and Equal Access in Social Care

Advocacy and equal access in social care are vital components of the support and services provided to individuals with disabilities.

These principles ensure that individuals receive equitable treatment and have their rights upheld in the context of social care.

Here is an overview of advocacy and equal access in social care in the UK, particularly for individuals with disabilities:

1. Addressing Disparities in Social Care:

- Advocacy in social care focuses on addressing disparities that individuals with disabilities may face in accessing social care services and support.

- These disparities can include difficulties in obtaining appropriate care, navigating the social care system or experiencing discrimination.

2. Legal Protections:

- The UK has legislation, such as the Equality Act 2010 and the Care Act 2014, which protect the rights of individuals with disabilities in social care settings.

- Advocates work to ensure that social care providers and local authorities adhere to these laws and provide accessible and equitable services.

3. Person-centred Approaches:

- Social care in the UK adopts person-centred approaches, which involve assessing and addressing the unique needs, preferences and goals of individuals with disabilities.

- Advocates promote these approaches to ensure that social care services are tailored to the individual.

4. Inclusive Services and Accommodations:

- Advocacy efforts encompass making social care services and accommodations inclusive and accessible to individuals with disabilities.

- This includes ensuring that care plans, care homes, day centres and supported living arrangements are designed to meet the needs of individuals with varying disabilities.

5. Support in Navigating the Social Care System:

- Advocates provide support to individuals with disabilities in navigating the complexities of the social care system.

- This assistance can include understanding eligibility criteria, making applications for support and appealing decisions.

6. Communication Accessibility:

- Advocacy emphasises the importance of effective communication between social care providers and individuals with disabilities.

- This may involve providing communication aids, sign language interpreters or accessible information formats.

7. Advocacy Services:

- Dedicated advocacy services provide individuals with disabilities with trained advocates who can represent their interests, help them voice their concerns and make informed choices about their social care.

8. Protection from Discrimination:

- Advocacy efforts are aimed at protecting individuals with disabilities from discrimination in social care settings.

- Advocates challenge discriminatory practices and attitudes that may hinder access to quality care.

9. Ensuring Accommodations:

- Advocates work to ensure that individuals with disabilities receive necessary accommodations to fully participate in social care decisions, activities and community engagement.

10. Promoting Inclusive Communities:

- Advocacy extends to promoting inclusive communities where individuals with disabilities can fully participate and engage in social activities, employment and community life.

11. Policy Change and Reform:

- Advocacy often involves advocating for policy changes and reforms in the social care sector to enhance access, improve care quality and protect the rights of individuals with disabilities.

12. Raising Awareness:

- Advocacy also includes raising awareness about the social care needs and challenges faced by individuals with disabilities in the UK, educating social care providers, local authorities and the public.

In summary, advocacy and equal access in social care in the UK for individuals with disabilities are essential for ensuring that they receive equitable and person-centred support.

These efforts encompass addressing disparities, ensuring legal protections, promoting accessibility, providing support in navigating the system, facilitating communication, combating discrimination and raising awareness.

Through advocacy and equal access initiatives, individuals with disabilities can access social care services that enhance their well-being and inclusion within the community.

Advocacy and Equal Access in Education (UK)

Advocacy and equal access are fundamental principles in the education sector in the United Kingdom, ensuring that students, including those with disabilities, have equitable opportunities for learning and personal development.

These principles promote an inclusive educational environment where all students can thrive.

Here is an overview of advocacy and equal access in education in the UK, particularly for students with disabilities:

1. Inclusive Education Policies:

- Advocacy efforts in education focus on the development and implementation of inclusive education policies that guarantee access to quality education for all students, regardless of their abilities or disabilities.

- These policies ensure that students with disabilities are not segregated from mainstream education.

2. Legal Frameworks:

- The UK has legal frameworks, including the Equality Act 2010 and the Children and Families Act 2014, which protect the rights of students with disabilities in educational settings.

- Advocates work to ensure that educational institutions adhere to these laws and provide reasonable accommodations.

3. Individualised Education Plans (IEPs):

- In the UK, students with disabilities often have Individualised Education Plans (IEPs) that outline their unique learning goals, accommodations and support services.

- Advocacy includes ensuring that IEPs are developed collaboratively with input from students, parents, educators and specialists.

4. Accessible Learning Environments:

- Advocacy efforts encompass making learning environments, including classrooms, curriculum materials and digital resources, accessible to all students.

- This includes providing accommodations such as assistive technology, accessible formats and accessible physical facilities.

5. Communication Accessibility:

- Advocacy emphasises effective communication between educators and students with disabilities.

- Schools provide communication aids, sign language interpreters or alternative communication methods as needed.

6. Support for Learning Needs:

- Advocates ensure that students with disabilities receive the necessary support to address their specific learning needs.

- This may involve additional teaching assistance, counselling or specialised instruction.

7. Transition Planning:

- Advocacy extends to planning for transitions in education, such as moving from primary to secondary school or transitioning to post-school life.

- Transition planning helps students with disabilities prepare for changes and ensures that their preferences and goals are considered.

8. Self-Advocacy Skills:

- Advocacy includes promoting self-advocacy skills among students with disabilities.

- These skills empower students to communicate their needs, seek accommodations and assert their rights.

9. Protection from Discrimination:

- Advocacy efforts are aimed at protecting students with disabilities from discrimination in educational settings.

- Advocates challenge discriminatory practices and attitudes that may hinder access to quality education.

10. Parental and Caregiver Advocacy:

- Parents and caregivers often play a critical role in advocating for the educational rights and needs of students with disabilities.

- Advocacy includes providing resources and support to parents in their advocacy efforts.

11. Raising Awareness:

- Advocacy also includes raising awareness about the educational needs and challenges faced by students with disabilities in the UK, educating educators, policymakers and the public.

12. Policy Change and Reform:

- Advocacy often involves advocating for policy changes and reforms in the education sector to enhance access, improve educational quality and protect the rights of students with disabilities.

In summary, advocacy and equal access in education in the UK for students with disabilities are essential for ensuring that they receive equitable educational opportunities and support.

These efforts encompass inclusive policies, legal protections, individualised plans, accessible environments, communication accessibility, learning support, transition planning, self-advocacy skills, protection from discrimination, parental advocacy, raising awareness and policy change initiatives.

Through advocacy and equal access initiatives, students with disabilities can access an inclusive education that promotes their personal growth and future success.

Advocacy and Equal Access in Childcare (UK)

Advocacy and equal access are essential principles in childcare in the United Kingdom, ensuring that all children, including those with disabilities, have the opportunity to access quality childcare services in an inclusive and equitable manner.

These principles promote an environment where children's rights and well-being are protected.

Here is an overview of advocacy and equal access in childcare in the UK, particularly for children with disabilities:

1. Inclusive Childcare Policies:

- Advocacy efforts in childcare focus on the development and implementation of inclusive childcare policies that ensure all children, regardless of their abilities or disabilities, have access to high-quality childcare services.

- These policies promote integrated childcare settings where children with disabilities can interact and learn alongside their typically developing peers.

2. Legal Protections:

- The UK has legal protections, including the Equality Act 2010, that safeguard the rights of children with disabilities in childcare settings.

- Advocates work to ensure that childcare providers and institutions adhere to these laws and provide appropriate accommodations.

3. Accessible Childcare Facilities:

- Advocacy includes making childcare facilities, both indoor and outdoor spaces, accessible to children with disabilities.

- This encompasses ensuring ramps, accessible restrooms and other accommodations to meet the diverse needs of children.

4. Inclusive Programming:

- Advocacy efforts focus on developing inclusive childcare programming that caters to the unique needs and interests of children with disabilities.

- This includes adapting activities, materials and learning environments to be accessible and engaging for all children.

5. Communication Accessibility:

- Advocacy emphasises effective communication between childcare providers and children with disabilities.

- This may involve providing communication aids, sign language interpreters or alternative communication methods.

6. Support for Diverse Learning Styles:

- Advocates work to ensure that childcare providers offer support for children with disabilities to meet their diverse learning styles and needs.

- Additional teaching assistance, specialised instruction or counselling may be provided as necessary.

7. Encouraging Children's Voices:

- Advocacy includes encouraging children with disabilities to have a say in their childcare experiences.

- This promotes their autonomy and fosters their self-esteem.

- Childcare providers create opportunities for children to make decisions about activities, playtime and routines.

8. Protection from Discrimination:

- Advocacy efforts are aimed at protecting children with disabilities from discrimination in childcare settings.

- Advocates challenge discriminatory practices and attitudes that may hinder access to quality childcare.

9. Parental and Caregiver Advocacy:

- Parents and caregivers often play a pivotal role in advocating for the rights and well-being of children with disabilities in childcare.

- Advocacy includes providing resources and support to parents and caregivers in their advocacy efforts.

10. Raising Awareness:

- Advocacy also includes raising awareness about the childcare needs and challenges faced by children with disabilities in the UK, educating childcare providers, policymakers and the public.

11. Policy Change and Reform:

- Advocacy often involves advocating for policy changes and reforms in the childcare sector to enhance access, improve childcare quality and protect the rights of children with disabilities.

In summary, advocacy and equal access in childcare in the

UK for children with disabilities are crucial for ensuring that they have the same opportunities for growth, development and social interaction as their peers.

These efforts encompass inclusive policies, legal protections, accessible facilities, inclusive programming, communication accessibility, learning support, encouraging children's voices, protection from discrimination, parental advocacy, raising awareness and policy change initiatives.

Through advocacy and equal access initiatives, children with disabilities can access childcare services that nurture their well-being and foster their development within inclusive and supportive environments.

7 SKILL BUILDING

Skill Building

Skill-building is a critical component of disability empowerment, as it equips individuals with disabilities with the knowledge, abilities and tools they need to live more independently and actively participate in their communities.

This process involves the acquisition and development of a range of skills that can enhance a person's self-confidence, self-reliance and overall quality of life.

Here are some key aspects of skill-building within the context of disability empowerment:

Communication Skills:

- Effective communication is essential for self-expression, social interaction and accessing support services.
- Skill-building in communication may include speech

therapy, sign language training or the use of augmentative and alternative communication (AAC) devices.

Problem-Solving Skills:

- Developing problem-solving skills empowers individuals to identify challenges, analyse them and work toward solutions.
- This skill is particularly valuable in navigating daily life and overcoming obstacles.

Self-Advocacy Skills:

- Self-advocacy involves speaking up for one's own needs and rights.
- Skill-building in self-advocacy helps individuals with disabilities become effective advocates for themselves, whether in healthcare settings, educational institutions or employment situations.

Daily Living Skills:

- These skills encompass a wide range of activities necessary for independent living, including personal hygiene, meal preparation, housekeeping and managing personal finances.
- Training in daily living skills promotes self-sufficiency.

Social Skills:

- Social interaction is an integral part of life.
- Skill-building in social skills helps individuals with disabilities develop meaningful relationships, engage

in social activities and navigate social norms and conventions.

Employment Skills:

- Acquiring job-related skills, such as resume writing, interview preparation and workplace etiquette, can enhance employability and facilitate access to meaningful employment opportunities.

Technology Skills:

- In today's digital world, technology proficiency is increasingly important.
- Skill-building in technology can include using assistive devices, accessing online resources and improving digital literacy.

Mobility and Transportation Skills:

- Learning to navigate public transportation or use mobility aids effectively is crucial for independence and community participation.
- Developing mobility and transportation skills not only enhances independence but also fosters social inclusion by enabling individuals with disabilities to access educational, employment, recreational and healthcare opportunities within their communities.

- These skills can encompass using mobility aids, understanding public transportation routes and learning safe practices for navigating various transportation modes.

Emotional Regulation and Coping Skills:

- Building emotional regulation and coping skills can help individuals with disabilities manage stress, anxiety and emotional challenges effectively.

Financial Literacy:

- Understanding financial concepts, budgeting and financial planning are important skills for managing personal finances and achieving financial independence.

Advocacy Skills:

- Beyond self-advocacy, advocacy skills can empower individuals to advocate for systemic changes that benefit the disability community as a whole.
- This may involve leadership training and community organising.

Educational Skills:

- For individuals pursuing education, skill-building may involve strategies for effective learning, time management and study skills.

Skill-building programs and interventions are often tailored to the specific needs and goals of each individual with a disability.

They can be delivered through various means, including one-on-one instruction, group training, educational programs and community-based services.

By acquiring these skills, individuals with disabilities can increase their independence, self-determination and overall quality of life, contributing to their empowerment and inclusion in society.

The Role of Healthcare Services in Skill Building and Education

Healthcare services play a multifaceted role in skill building and education, extending beyond traditional medical treatment to support individuals in acquiring essential life skills and knowledge.

This holistic approach to healthcare recognises that a person's well-being is influenced by factors beyond their physical health, including their ability to function independently and engage in educational pursuits.

Here's how healthcare services can contribute to skill building and education, promoting disability empowerment:

1. Rehabilitation Services:

- Healthcare services, particularly rehabilitation programs, help individuals recover from injuries or illnesses that may have affected their physical or cognitive abilities.

- Rehabilitation therapists work with patients to regain mobility, speech and cognitive functions, enabling them to participate in educational and vocational activities.

2. Pediatric Developmental Services:

- For children with developmental delays or

disabilities, healthcare services often include early intervention programs.

- These programs focus on developing essential skills in areas such as communication, fine and gross motor skills and cognitive abilities to prepare children for educational settings.

3. Specialised Training and Therapy:

- Healthcare professionals, such as occupational therapists and speech-language pathologists, provide specialised training and therapy to individuals with disabilities.

- This includes teaching communication skills, mobility techniques and adaptive strategies that enhance a person's ability to participate in educational settings.

4. Mental Health and Behavioral Support:

- Mental health services offer counselling and support to individuals dealing with emotional or behavioural challenges.

- Addressing mental health concerns is essential for a person's well-being and their ability to engage effectively in educational and social environments.

5. Assistive Technology and Devices:

- Healthcare services include the assessment and provision of assistive technology and devices.

- These technologies, such as communication devices, mobility aids and adaptive software, enable individuals with disabilities to access educational resources and participate in learning activities.

6. Health Education:

- Healthcare providers offer health education to individuals and families, promoting a better understanding of medical conditions and their management.

- Health literacy is a foundational skill that contributes to informed decision-making and self-advocacy, which are crucial in educational settings.

7. Preventive Care and Well-Being:

- Preventive healthcare services, such as vaccinations and wellness check-ups, support individuals in maintaining good health.

- Being in good health is a prerequisite for effective learning and skill development.

8. Coordination of Care:

- Healthcare services often involve care coordination, where healthcare professionals collaborate with educators, therapists and caregivers.

- This coordination ensures that a person's healthcare needs align with their educational goals and support their overall development.

9. Transition Planning:

- Healthcare services can assist individuals with disabilities in transitioning from paediatric to adult care.

- Transition planning addresses both healthcare and educational needs as young adults prepare for independent living and continued education.

10. Parent and Caregiver Education:

- Healthcare services provide education and guidance to parents and caregivers, empowering them to support their loved ones in skill building and education.

- Informed caregivers play a vital role in a person's educational journey.

11. Community Resources and Referrals:

- Healthcare providers often connect individuals and families with community resources, including educational support services, vocational training programs and advocacy organisations.

- These resources enhance access to education and skill-building opportunities.

In summary, healthcare services contribute significantly to skill building and education by addressing physical, cognitive and emotional needs.

Through rehabilitation, therapy, assistive technology, health education and collaboration with other professionals, healthcare services support individuals in achieving their educational goals and developing essential life skills.

This holistic approach to healthcare recognises that well-rounded support is essential for individuals to thrive academically and personally.

The Role of Social Care Services in Skill Building and Education

Social care services play a pivotal role in skill building and education by providing individuals, especially those with disabilities or specific needs, with the necessary support and resources to enhance their abilities, access education and participate fully in society.

Here's how social care services can contribute to skill building and education, promoting disability empowerment:

1. Personalised Support Plans:

- Social care services create personalised support plans that address the unique needs and goals of individuals.

- These plans often include educational and skill development objectives.

2. Inclusive Care Settings:

- Social care services aim to create inclusive environments where individuals can interact with their peers, build social skills and access educational opportunities.

- This inclusivity is particularly beneficial for children and adults with disabilities, as it promotes social interaction and learning.

3. Support for Daily Living Skills:

- Social care providers assist individuals in developing

essential daily living skills, such as personal hygiene, meal preparation and household management.

- These skills enhance a person's independence and readiness for educational settings.

4. Assistance with Homework and Learning Activities:

- For children and young people, social care services often provide assistance with homework, learning activities and educational support.

- This ensures that they can keep up with their peers in school.

5. Communication and Socialisation Support:

- Social care services offer communication and socialisation support for individuals who may struggle with these aspects.

- This support can include speech therapy, social skills training and peer interaction programs.

6. Access to Specialist Services:

- Social care services can connect individuals with disabilities to specialist services and therapists who can address specific learning or developmental challenges.

- This ensures that the educational needs of the individual are met.

7. Transition Planning:

- Social care services often assist young adults with disabilities in transitioning from school to further education or employment.

- Transition planning helps individuals identify their goals and access the necessary resources and support.

8. Respite Care for Caregivers:

- Social care services provide respite care for family caregivers, giving them the opportunity to engage in educational activities or seek further education themselves.

9. Support for Lifelong Learning:

- Social care services recognise that education is a lifelong process. They support individuals in pursuing further education or skill development at any stage of life.

10. Advocacy and Rights Protection:

- Social care providers often act as advocates for individuals with disabilities, ensuring that they have equal access to educational opportunities and that their rights are protected.

11. Coordination with Educational Providers:

- Social care services collaborate with educational institutions to ensure that the support provided aligns with a person's educational goals.

- This coordination can involve sharing information and creating strategies to facilitate learning.

12. Building Independence:

- Social care services empower individuals to develop independence by teaching skills related to mobility, decision-making and self-advocacy.

- Independence is a fundamental skill that supports lifelong learning.

13. Emotional and Behavioral Support:

- Social care services address emotional and behavioural challenges that may impact an individual's ability to learn and engage in education.

- This support contributes to a conducive learning environment.

In summary, social care services play a crucial role in skill building and education by providing tailored support, fostering inclusivity, assisting with daily living skills, facilitating access to specialist services, promoting independence and advocating for individuals with disabilities.

Through these efforts, social care services empower individuals to achieve their educational goals and build essential life skills, ensuring that they can participate fully in education and society.

The Role of Residential Care Settings in Skill Building and Education

Residential care settings, such as care homes and group homes, serve as crucial environments for individuals who require support and assistance due to various challenges, including disabilities and age-related needs.

These settings play a significant role in skill building and education, focusing on the well-being and development of residents.

Here's how residential care settings can contribute to skill building and education, promoting disability awareness:

1. Individualised Care Plans:

- Residential care settings develop individualised care plans for each resident, which include educational and skill-building components.

- These plans are tailored to the unique needs and goals of residents, whether they are children, young adults or seniors.

2. Specialised Programs:

- Many residential care settings offer specialised programs and activities designed to enhance residents' cognitive, physical and social abilities.

- These programs may include educational workshops, physical therapy, art therapy and more.

3. Access to Educational Resources:

- Residential care settings ensure that residents have access to educational resources, including books, computers and educational materials.

- This support enables residents to engage in self-directed learning and explore their interests.

4. Life Skills Development:

- Residential care staff work with residents to develop essential life skills, such as cooking, cleaning, personal hygiene and budgeting.

- These skills promote independence and self-sufficiency.

5. Support for Homework and Academic Pursuits:

- For children and young adults in residential care, staff often provide assistance with homework, educational projects and academic pursuits.

- This support helps them excel academically.

6. Transition Planning:

- Residential care settings assist young adults in transitioning to independent living, vocational training or further education.

- Transition planning ensures that residents are prepared for the next phase of their lives.

7. Emotional and Behavioral Support:

- Staff in residential care settings address emotional and behavioural challenges by providing counselling and therapeutic interventions.

- Emotional well-being is essential for effective learning and skill development.

8. Accessible Facilities:

- Residential care settings are equipped with accessible facilities to accommodate the needs of residents with disabilities.

- This includes ramps, wide doorways and adapted bathrooms.

9. Health and Nutrition Education:

- Many residential care settings offer health and nutrition education to residents, promoting healthy lifestyle choices and well-being.

10. Recreational and Social Activities:

- Social interaction and recreational activities, such as group outings and community events, are integral components of residential care settings.

- These activities enhance social skills and community engagement.

11. Vocational Training:

- Some residential care settings provide vocational training opportunities, equipping residents with job-related skills and knowledge.

- This prepares them for employment and self-sufficiency.

12. Advocacy and Rights Protection:

- Staff in residential care settings act as advocates for residents, ensuring that they have equal access to educational opportunities and that their rights are protected.

13. Family and Caregiver Engagement:

- Residential care settings involve families and caregivers in the care and education of residents.

- Collaboration ensures a holistic approach to residents' development.

14. Independence and Self-Advocacy:

- Residential care promotes residents' independence by teaching mobility skills, self-advocacy and decision-making.

- These skills are valuable for lifelong learning and personal growth.

In summary, residential care settings are essential in skill building and education, providing individualised care plans, specialised programs, educational resources, life skills development, academic support, transition planning, emotional and behavioural support, accessible facilities, health education, recreational activities, vocational training, advocacy, family engagement and the promotion of independence.

Through these efforts, residents in care settings can enhance their abilities, pursue educational goals and lead fulfilling lives within a supportive and inclusive environment.

The Role of Education Services in Skill Building and Education

Education services encompass a wide range of formal and informal learning opportunities provided by schools, colleges, universities and community organisations.

These services play a central role in skill building and education for individuals of all ages and backgrounds.

Here's how education services can contribute to skill building and education, promoting disability empowerment:

1. Formal Education Programs:

- Schools, colleges and universities offer formal education programs that provide structured curricula and academic instruction.

- These programs equip students with foundational knowledge and skills, including reading, writing, mathematics and critical thinking.

2. Special Education Programs:

- Special education programs within schools cater to the unique needs of students with disabilities.

- They offer tailored instruction, accommodations and support services to help these students succeed academically and develop essential life skills.

3. Vocational and Technical Training:

- Vocational schools and technical training programs offer specialised training in trades, technology and specific industries.

- This training prepares individuals for careers and equips them with practical skills.

4. Adult and Continuing Education:

- Adult education programs and lifelong learning opportunities allow individuals to acquire new skills and knowledge throughout their lives.

- These programs support career advancement, personal enrichment and skill development.

5. Distance and Online Learning:

- Distance and online learning options provide flexibility for individuals who may have constraints on attending traditional classes.

- They offer a wide range of courses and programs accessible from anywhere with an internet connection.

6. Inclusive Education:

- Inclusive education policies promote diversity and accommodate students with disabilities within mainstream classrooms.

- Inclusion fosters social interaction, tolerance and the development of social and emotional skills.

7. Extracurricular Activities:

- Extracurricular activities, such as sports, clubs and arts programs, complement formal education.

- They help students develop teamwork, leadership and creative skills.

8. Career Counselling and Guidance:

- Educational institutions often provide career counselling services to help students explore career options and plan their educational paths.

- Career guidance supports informed decision-making.

9. Specialised Support Services:

- Education services may offer specialised support services, including tutoring, counselling and academic accommodations, to assist students with diverse needs.

- These services ensure that all students have an equal opportunity to succeed.

10. Inclusive and Accessible Learning Environments:

- Schools and educational institutions work to create inclusive and accessible learning environments.

- This includes physical accessibility, adaptive

technologies and support for students with disabilities.

11. Professional Development:

- Education services extend to professional development programs for educators, enabling them to enhance their teaching skills and stay updated on best practices.

12. Community Education:

- Community organisations often provide educational programs that address local needs and interests.

- These programs promote community engagement and skill development.

13. Education for Personal Growth:

- Education services acknowledge the importance of personal growth and self-improvement.

- Lifelong learning opportunities allow individuals to pursue interests and hobbies.

14. Advocacy for Educational Rights:

- Education services may advocate for the rights of students, particularly those with disabilities, to ensure equal access to educational opportunities.

15. Collaboration with Other Services:

- Education services often collaborate with healthcare, social care and vocational services to provide comprehensive support to individuals with complex needs.

In summary, education services are essential for skill building and education, offering formal and specialised programs, vocational training, adult and continuing education, distance learning, inclusive education, extracurricular activities, career counselling, support services, accessible environments, professional development, community education, personal growth opportunities, advocacy and collaborative efforts.

Through these services, individuals can acquire knowledge, develop skills and achieve their educational and personal goals, leading to enhanced opportunities and well-rounded development.

The Role of Childcare Services in Skill Building and Education

Childcare services are crucial in providing a safe, nurturing environment for young children while also supporting their early skill building and educational development.

These services encompass a range of settings, from home-based childcare to formal preschools and daycare centres.

Here's how childcare services can contribute to skill building and education for young children, promoting disability empowerment:

1. Early Learning and School Readiness:

- Childcare services often incorporate early learning programs that introduce children to foundational skills such as language development, pre-mathematics and social interaction.

- These programs help prepare children for formal schooling.

2. Cognitive and Language Development:

- Childcare providers engage children in activities that stimulate cognitive and language development.

- Through storytelling, play and educational games, children acquire essential skills for communication and problem-solving.

3. Socialisation and Emotional Development:

- Childcare settings promote socialisation and emotional development by encouraging interactions with peers and adults.

- Children learn essential skills like sharing, empathy and conflict resolution.

4. Play-Based Learning:

- Play is a fundamental aspect of early childhood education.

- Childcare services incorporate play-based learning, where children explore their creativity and problem-solving abilities.

- Play activities foster skill development in areas like motor skills, imagination and critical thinking.

5. Early Literacy and Numeracy Skills:

- Childcare providers introduce early literacy and numeracy concepts through age-appropriate activities.

- These activities lay the foundation for reading, writing and mathematics.

6. Multicultural and Inclusive Education:

- Many childcare services embrace diversity and

inclusivity by introducing children to various cultures, languages and abilities.

- This promotes tolerance and appreciation of differences.

7. Structured Educational Programs:

- Some childcare centres offer structured educational programs that follow curricula designed to enhance children's educational and developmental progress.

- These programs provide a structured learning environment.

8. Health and Safety Education:

- Childcare services teach children about health and safety topics, including personal hygiene, nutrition and emergency procedures.

- These lessons contribute to overall well-being.

9. Parent Engagement:

- Childcare providers often involve parents in their child's educational journey by sharing progress reports, offering parent-teacher conferences and suggesting activities for home learning.

10. Early Intervention:

- Childcare services may identify developmental delays or challenges early on and collaborate with families to access early intervention services and support.

11. Language Exposure:

- In multicultural settings, childcare services expose

children to a variety of languages, promoting language development and cultural awareness.

12. Preparation for School Transition:

- Childcare services help children transition smoothly into formal schooling by familiarising them with routines, structure and educational concepts.

13. Observation and Assessment:

- Childcare providers observe and assess children's developmental progress, identifying areas where additional support may be needed.

14. Individualised Support:

- Childcare professionals offer individualised support to children with special needs, ensuring that they receive the necessary accommodations and assistance.

15. Encouragement of Curiosity:

- Childcare services foster a love for learning by encouraging children's natural curiosity and exploration.

The Role of Childcare Services in Disability Empowerment through Skill Building and Education

Childcare services are instrumental in promoting disability empowerment by providing young children with disabilities a supportive and inclusive environment for skill building and education.

These services contribute significantly to fostering independence, self-esteem and a strong foundation for lifelong learning.

Here's how childcare services can play a pivotal role in disability empowerment through skill building and education:

1. Inclusive Environments:

- Childcare services promote inclusive environments where children with disabilities are integrated with their peers.

- Inclusion allows children to learn from one another and fosters empathy, tolerance and acceptance.

2. Individualised Support Plans:

- Childcare providers work closely with families to create individualised support plans for children with disabilities.

- These plans address specific educational goals, accommodations and interventions tailored to the child's unique needs.

3. Early Intervention and Assessment:

- Childcare services often collaborate with early intervention professionals to identify developmental delays or disabilities in young children.

- Early assessment and support help address challenges proactively.

4. Adaptive Equipment and Technology:

- Childcare providers ensure that children with disabilities have access to adaptive equipment and assistive technology that facilitate their participation in educational activities.

- These tools empower children to engage effectively in learning experiences.

5. Communication Support:

- Childcare staff are trained to provide communication support to children with speech or language impairments.

- This support helps children express themselves and communicate with peers and caregivers.

6. Social Skills and Peer Interaction:

- Childcare services prioritise social skills development, fostering peer interactions and friendships among children with and without disabilities.

- These interactions contribute to emotional growth and self-confidence.

7. Play-Based Learning:

- Play-based learning is a cornerstone of childcare services, allowing children with disabilities to explore and develop their motor, cognitive and imaginative skills.
- Play activities are adapted to accommodate individual needs.

8. Sensory Integration:

- Childcare providers incorporate sensory integration activities to support children with sensory processing challenges.

- These activities help children regulate their sensory

experiences and engage in learning.

9. Positive Reinforcement and Self-Esteem Building:

- Childcare professionals focus on positive reinforcement and building self-esteem in children with disabilities.

- Encouraging achievements and highlighting strengths contribute to a positive self-image.

10. Collaboration with Specialists:

- Childcare services collaborate with specialists such as speech therapists, occupational therapists and behaviour analysts to provide targeted support.

- This multidisciplinary approach addresses a wide range of needs.

11. Family Involvement:

- Childcare providers actively involve families in the child's educational journey.

- Parents and caregivers are informed, engaged and empowered to support their child's skill development.

12. Transition Planning:

- Childcare services assist in the transition from childcare to formal education, ensuring that children with disabilities are well-prepared for the next educational phase.

13. Advocacy and Rights Awareness:

- Childcare providers educate families about the rights and resources available to children with disabilities.

- Advocacy efforts empower families to navigate the education system effectively.

14. Emphasis on Abilities:

- Childcare services emphasise children's abilities rather than focusing on their disabilities.

- This approach fosters a positive attitude and encourages children to reach their full potential.

In summary, childcare services play a vital role in disability empowerment through skill building and education by promoting inclusive environments, providing individualised support, facilitating early intervention, offering adaptive equipment and technology, supporting communication, fostering social skills, emphasising play-based learning, addressing sensory needs, building self-esteem, collaborating with specialists, engaging families, assisting with transitions, raising awareness of rights and highlighting children's abilities.

These efforts empower children with disabilities to thrive, learn and develop a strong foundation for a future of opportunities.

8 POSITIVE SELF-IMAGE AND PRIDE

Positive Self-Image

Fostering a positive self-image and promoting self-esteem among individuals with disabilities is a critical aspect of disability empowerment. This process involves challenging stereotypes, combating discrimination and cultivating a sense of pride and self-worth.

Here's why positive self-image is essential and how it can be encouraged:

Self-Confidence:

- Positive self-image boosts self-confidence.
- When individuals with disabilities believe in their abilities and worth, they are more likely to pursue their goals and aspirations with determination.

Self-Acceptance:

- Encouraging a positive self-image helps individuals accept themselves as they are, recognising that disability is just one aspect of their identity.
- This acceptance fosters a sense of belonging and

self-compassion.

Overcoming Stereotypes:

- Society often perpetuates negative stereotypes about people with disabilities.
- Promoting a positive self-image challenges these stereotypes by emphasising the diverse talents, skills and capabilities of individuals with disabilities.

Resilience:

- Individuals with a positive self-image are more resilient in the face of challenges and adversity.
- They are better equipped to cope with discrimination, setbacks and obstacles.

Advocacy:

- People with disabilities who have a strong sense of self-worth are more likely to advocate for themselves and their rights.
- They are also more effective advocates for broader social change.

Social Inclusion:

- Positive self-image contributes to social inclusion.
- Individuals who feel good about themselves are more likely to engage in social activities, build relationships and participate in their communities.

Reducing Stigma:

- A positive self-image can help reduce the stigma associated with disabilities.
- When people with disabilities are confident and proud of who they are, it challenges negative attitudes and perceptions held by others.

Empowerment:

- Empowerment begins with a belief in one's own capacity to effect change.
- A positive self-image empowers individuals to take control of their lives, make decisions and pursue their goals.

Ways to Encourage Positive Self-Image in Individuals with Disabilities:

Promote Inclusive Education:

- Inclusive education environments that value diversity and celebrate individual achievements can boost self-esteem among students with disabilities.

Highlight Strengths:

- Emphasise and celebrate the unique strengths, talents and accomplishments of individuals with disabilities.
- Recognise and showcase their contributions to their communities.

Provide Role Models:

- Share stories and examples of successful individuals with disabilities who have achieved their goals and made significant contributions to society.

- Role models can inspire and provide hope.

Offer Support:

- Provide emotional support and create safe spaces where individuals with disabilities can express themselves, share their experiences and seek guidance without fear of judgment.

Encourage Self-Advocacy:

- Teach self-advocacy skills, empowering individuals to assert their rights, express their needs and advocate for themselves.

Celebrate Achievements:

- Celebrate achievements and milestones, no matter how small they may seem. Recognition can boost self-esteem and motivation.

Challenge Negative Messages:

- Be vigilant in challenging negative messages and attitudes toward disability, both within the community and in media portrayals.

Encourage Independence:

- Encourage individuals with disabilities to be as independent as possible, allowing them to build a sense of self-efficacy and accomplishment.

Provide Positive Feedback:

- Offer positive feedback and constructive encouragement, reinforcing the idea that individuals with disabilities are valued members of their communities.

Promote Self-Reflection:

- Encourage self-reflection and self-awareness, helping individuals understand their strengths, values and aspirations.

Cultivate a Supportive Network:

- Build and nurture supportive networks that offer encouragement and affirmation, whether through peer support groups, mentors or family and friends.

By fostering a positive self-image and self-esteem, disability empowerment efforts can help individuals with disabilities realise their full potential, lead fulfilling lives and actively contribute to their communities. This, in turn, promotes a more inclusive and accepting society.

The Role of Healthcare Services in Fostering a Positive Self-Image and Pride in Disability Empowerment

Healthcare services play a crucial role in promoting disability empowerment by not only addressing medical needs but also nurturing a positive self-image and fostering a sense of pride among individuals with disabilities.

This holistic approach to care enhances overall well-being and self-worth.

Here's how healthcare services can contribute to fostering a positive self-image and pride in disability empowerment:

1. Comprehensive Healthcare Support:

- Healthcare services provide individuals with disabilities access to comprehensive care that addresses their physical, emotional and psychological well-being.

- This holistic approach recognises that well-rounded health contributes to a positive self-image.

2. Rehabilitation and Therapy:

- Rehabilitation services, including physical therapy, occupational therapy and speech therapy, support individuals in regaining or improving their physical abilities.
- Achieving functional goals enhances self-esteem and pride in one's accomplishments.

3. Pain Management and Comfort:

- Healthcare professionals prioritise pain management and comfort for individuals with chronic conditions or disabilities.

- This focus on well-being contributes to a positive outlook on life.

4. Mental Health Support:

- Healthcare services often include mental health support for individuals with disabilities who may experience depression, anxiety or other emotional challenges.

- Addressing mental health is essential for self-esteem and overall empowerment.

5. Support for Coping and Adjustment:

- Healthcare providers offer counselling and support to individuals and their families as they navigate the emotional and psychological aspects of disability.

- This support helps individuals build resilience and adapt positively to their circumstances.

6. Adaptive Devices and Technology:

- Healthcare services assist individuals in obtaining adaptive devices and assistive technology that enhance their independence and quality of life.

- These tools promote a sense of self-sufficiency and pride in one's abilities.

7. Education and Information Sharing:

- Healthcare professionals educate individuals with disabilities about their conditions, treatment options and self-care strategies.

- Informed individuals are better equipped to manage their health, leading to greater self-confidence.

8. Peer Support and Group Therapy:

- Many healthcare services offer peer support groups and group therapy sessions where individuals with similar challenges can connect, share experiences and build a sense of community.

- These interactions boost self-esteem and reduce feelings of isolation.

9. Empowerment-Based Care Plans:

- Healthcare providers collaborate with individuals to create care plans that emphasise their strengths, goals and aspirations.

- This empowerment-based approach promotes a positive self-image.

10. Advocacy for Inclusive Healthcare:

- Healthcare services advocate for inclusive

healthcare practices that consider the unique needs and preferences of individuals with disabilities.

- Ensuring equal access to healthcare services bolsters self-worth and pride.

11. Promoting Body Positivity:

- Healthcare professionals promote body positivity and self-acceptance, emphasising that individuals with disabilities are valuable and beautiful as they are.

- This perspective enhances self-esteem and self-image.

12. Celebrating Achievements:

- Healthcare providers celebrate individuals' achievements, whether they are related to improved health outcomes or personal milestones.

- Acknowledging accomplishments boosts pride and self-worth.

13. Encouraging Self-Advocacy:

- Healthcare services empower individuals with disabilities to advocate for themselves in healthcare decision-making.

- Self-advocacy promotes a sense of control and pride in one's ability to make informed choices.

14. Cultural Competence:

- Healthcare providers undergo cultural competence training to ensure that they respect the diverse backgrounds and identities of individuals with disabilities.

- This fosters a sense of belonging and pride in one's

identity.

In summary, healthcare services can contribute significantly to disability empowerment by providing comprehensive support, rehabilitation, mental health care, adaptive technology, education, peer support, empowerment-based care, advocacy, body positivity, celebration of achievements, self-advocacy encouragement, cultural competence and a focus on holistic well-being.

Through these efforts, individuals with disabilities can develop a positive self-image, feel pride in their accomplishments and lead fulfilling lives with a strong sense of self-worth.

The Role of Social Care Services in Fostering a Positive Self-Image and Pride in Disability Empowerment

Social care services are pivotal in disability empowerment, as they provide individuals with disabilities the support and tools needed to develop a positive self-image and take pride in their unique abilities.

These services focus on enhancing self-esteem, self-worth and a sense of belonging within the community.

Here's how social care services can contribute to fostering a positive self-image and pride in disability empowerment:

1. Person-centred Support:

- Social care services emphasise person-centred care, tailoring support plans to meet the specific needs, preferences and aspirations of each individual.

- This personalised approach empowers individuals to

take charge of their lives and boosts their self-esteem.

2. Inclusive Community Engagement:

- Social care providers encourage active participation in community activities, promoting social inclusion and reducing feelings of isolation.
- Engagement in community life fosters a sense of belonging and pride in one's contributions.

3. Peer Support Groups:

- Social care services facilitate peer support groups, where individuals with disabilities can connect, share experiences and offer mutual encouragement.

- These groups provide a platform for building relationships and boosting self-confidence.

4. Skill Development and Independence:

- Social care programs often focus on skill development, equipping individuals with essential life skills such as communication, problem-solving and daily living skills.

- Gaining these skills enhances independence and self-worth.

5. Self-Advocacy Training:

- Social care services empower individuals to become self-advocates, teaching them how to assert their needs and rights.

- Advocacy skills build self-confidence and a sense of agency.

6. Support for Emotional Well-Being:

- Social care providers offer emotional support and counselling to help individuals cope with the emotional challenges they may face.

- Addressing emotional well-being is essential for a positive self-image.

7. Accessible Community Resources:

- Social care services assist individuals in accessing community resources, including accessible transportation, housing and recreational activities.

- Ensuring accessibility promotes a sense of belonging and inclusion.

8. Celebrating Achievements:

- Social care professionals celebrate individuals' achievements, whether they are related to personal goals, employment or community involvement.

- Recognising accomplishments boosts self-esteem and pride.

9. Encouragement of Interests and Hobbies:

- Social care services encourage individuals to explore their interests and hobbies, fostering a sense of passion and purpose.

- Pursuing interests contributes to a positive self-image.

10. Advocacy for Equal Opportunities:

- Social care providers often engage in advocacy

efforts to ensure that individuals with disabilities have equal access to services, employment, education and other opportunities.

- Advocacy reinforces a sense of belonging and empowerment.

11. Cultural Sensitivity:

- Social care services prioritise cultural sensitivity and respect for the diverse backgrounds and identities of individuals with disabilities.

- This approach fosters pride in one's cultural heritage and identity.

12. Positive Role Models:

- Social care providers introduce individuals to positive role models with disabilities who have achieved success in various fields.

- These role models inspire individuals and instil a sense of possibility and pride.

13. Encouragement of Self-Expression:

- Social care services support individuals in expressing themselves through art, music, writing or other creative outlets.

- Self-expression fosters self-discovery and a positive self-image.

In summary, social care services can contribute significantly to disability empowerment by offering person-centred support, promoting community engagement, facilitating peer support, developing essential life skills, teaching self-advocacy, addressing emotional well-being, ensuring accessibility, celebrating achievements, encouraging interests and hobbies, advocating for equal opportunities, embracing cultural sensitivity, presenting positive role models and encouraging self-expression.

Through these efforts, individuals with disabilities can develop a strong sense of self-worth, pride in their accomplishments and a positive self-image that empowers them to lead fulfilling lives.

The Role of Residential Care Services in Fostering a Positive Self-Image and Pride in Disability Empowerment

Residential care services, including care homes and group homes, play a pivotal role in disability empowerment by providing a supportive and inclusive environment where individuals with disabilities can develop a positive self-image and take pride in their unique abilities.

These services focus on enhancing self-esteem, self-worth and overall well-being.

Here's how residential care services can contribute to fostering a positive self-image and pride in disability empowerment:

1. Individualised Care and Support:

- Residential care services prioritise individualised care plans tailored to each resident's specific needs, preferences and aspirations.

- This personalised approach empowers residents to actively participate in decisions regarding their care, enhancing their self-esteem and sense of agency.

2. Inclusive and Supportive Communities:

- Residential care settings foster inclusive and supportive communities where residents with disabilities live alongside their peers.

- This environment promotes social inclusion, reduces isolation and boosts residents' sense of belonging and pride in their community.

3. Skill-Building Programs:

- Many residential care services offer skill-building programs that help residents acquire essential life skills, such as cooking, cleaning and personal hygiene.

- Gaining these skills enhances residents' independence and self-worth.

4. Encouragement of Personal Interests and Hobbies:

- Residential care providers encourage residents to pursue their personal interests and hobbies, fostering a sense of passion and purpose.

- Pursuing individual interests contributes to a positive self-image.

5. Emotional and Behavioral Support:

- Residential care staff provide emotional and behavioural support to help residents cope with challenges and develop effective coping strategies.

- Addressing emotional well-being is crucial for self-esteem and empowerment.

6. Peer Support and Community Engagement:

- Residential care settings facilitate peer support and

community engagement through group activities, outings and shared living spaces.

- Residents can build friendships, share experiences and develop a sense of pride in their social connections.

7. Independence and Self-Advocacy Training:

- Residential care services focus on equipping residents with the skills needed to lead more independent lives and become self-advocates.
- Empowering residents with these skills boosts their self-confidence and self-worth.

8. Celebrating Achievements:

- Residential care professionals celebrate residents' accomplishments, whether related to personal goals, employment or community involvement.

- Recognising achievements fosters self-esteem and pride.

9. Cultural Sensitivity and Inclusivity:

- Residential care providers prioritise cultural sensitivity and embrace diversity within their communities.

- This approach fosters pride in one's cultural heritage and identity.

10. Access to Supportive Services:

- Residents have access to supportive services, including healthcare, therapy and vocational training, within the residential care setting.

- These services empower residents to lead fulfilling

lives with the necessary support.

11. Encouragement of Self-Expression:

- Residential care services support residents in expressing themselves through creative outlets such as art, music and writing.

- Self-expression contributes to self-discovery and a positive self-image.

12. Independence in Daily Living:

- Residential care staff work with residents to develop independence in daily living activities, such as managing personal finances and transportation.

- This autonomy boosts self-esteem.

In summary, residential care services contribute can significantly to disability empowerment by providing individualised care and support, fostering inclusive communities, offering skill-building programs, encouraging personal interests and hobbies, providing emotional and behavioural support, promoting peer support and community engagement, teaching independence and self-advocacy, celebrating achievements, embracing cultural sensitivity, offering supportive services and encouraging self-expression.

Through these efforts, individuals with disabilities in residential care can develop a strong sense of self-worth, pride in their accomplishments and a positive self-image that empowers them to live meaningful and fulfilling lives.

The Role of Education Services in Fostering a Positive Self-Image and Pride in Disability Empowerment

Education services play a pivotal role in disability empowerment by providing individuals with disabilities the opportunity to learn, grow and develop a positive self-image.

These services emphasise the importance of embracing one's unique abilities and achievements.

Here's how education services can contribute to fostering a positive self-image and pride in disability empowerment:

1. Inclusive and Accessible Learning Environments:

- Education services strive to create inclusive and accessible learning environments where students with disabilities can participate fully.

- Inclusion promotes a sense of belonging and pride in being part of the educational community.

2. Individualised Education Plans (IEPs):

- Students with disabilities often have Individualised Education Plans (IEPs) that outline personalised goals, accommodations and support.

- IEPs empower students to take an active role in their education and set achievable objectives.

3. Supportive Teachers and Staff:

- Educators and support staff in educational settings receive training in supporting students with disabilities.

- Their commitment and support contribute to students' self-esteem and self-worth.

4. Celebrating Achievements:

- Education services celebrate students' accomplishments, both academically and personally.

- Recognising achievements fosters self-esteem and pride.

5. Encouragement of Ambitions:

- Education professionals encourage students to pursue their ambitions and interests.
- This encouragement instils a sense of passion and purpose.

6. Peer Relationships and Social Skills:

- Educational settings provide opportunities for students to develop peer relationships and social skills.

- Building friendships and social connections boosts students' sense of belonging and self-worth.

7. Inclusive Curriculum:

- Curriculum designers in education services work to create inclusive educational materials and resources.

- Inclusive materials promote diversity and allow students to see themselves represented positively.

8. Emphasis on Strengths:

- Education services focus on identifying and nurturing students' strengths rather than solely addressing weaknesses.

- This approach encourages students to take pride in their unique abilities.

9. Access to Assistive Technology:

- Students with disabilities have access to assistive technology and tools that enable them to engage fully in educational activities.

- Assistive technology promotes independence and self-worth.

10. Peer Mentoring Programs:

- Some educational institutions establish peer mentoring programs where students with disabilities can mentor and support one another.

- Peer mentoring builds a sense of community and empowerment.

11. Inclusive Extracurricular Activities:

- Education services offer inclusive extracurricular activities that allow students to explore their interests and passions.

- Participation in 'extracurriculars' enhances self-esteem.

12. Access to Supportive Services:

- Education services may provide access to supportive services, such as counselling or therapy, to address emotional and psychological needs.

- Emotional well-being is essential for self-esteem and empowerment.

13. Self-Advocacy Skills:

- Students are taught self-advocacy skills, empowering them to communicate their needs and preferences in the educational setting.

- Self-advocacy builds self-confidence and a sense of agency.

14. Transition Planning:

- Education services assist students in transition planning for life beyond school, including post-secondary education or employment.

- This planning reinforces a sense of hope and purpose.

In summary, education services contribute significantly to disability empowerment by creating inclusive learning environments, offering individualised education plans, providing supportive staff, celebrating achievements, encouraging ambitions, fostering peer relationships, emphasising strengths, offering assistive technology, implementing peer mentoring programs, providing inclusive extracurricular activities, granting access to supportive services, teaching self-advocacy skills and assisting with transition planning.

Through these efforts, individuals with disabilities in educational settings can develop a strong sense of self-worth, pride in their accomplishments and a positive self-image that empowers them to pursue their dreams and contribute to society.

The Role of Childcare Services in Fostering a Positive Self-Image and Pride in Disability Empowerment

Childcare services are instrumental in disability empowerment, as they provide young children with disabilities a nurturing and inclusive environment where they can develop a positive self-image and take pride in their unique abilities.

These services lay the foundation for self-esteem, self-worth and a sense of belonging.

Here's how childcare services can contribute to fostering a positive self-image and pride in disability empowerment:

1. Inclusive Play and Learning:

- Childcare services promote inclusive play and learning experiences where children with disabilities interact with their peers.

- Inclusive activities build a sense of belonging and pride in being part of the group.

2. Individualised Support:

- Childcare providers create individualised support plans that address the specific needs and preferences of each child with a disability.

- Individualisation empowers children and recognises their uniqueness.

3. Early Intervention and Early Learning:

- Childcare settings often collaborate with early intervention specialists to identify developmental delays and provide early support.

- Early learning opportunities contribute to positive self-image.

4. Adaptive Toys and Equipment:

- Childcare services ensure that children with disabilities have access to adaptive toys and equipment that facilitate their participation.

- These tools promote independence and self-worth.

5. Communication Support:

- Childcare staff are trained to provide communication support to children with speech or language impairments.

- Improved communication enhances self-esteem and self-expression.

6. Positive Reinforcement:

- Childcare providers use positive reinforcement to acknowledge children's efforts and accomplishments.

- Positive feedback boosts self-esteem and pride.

7. Sensory Integration Activities:

- Childcare services incorporate sensory integration activities that help children with sensory processing challenges.

- Sensory activities support self-regulation and engagement.

8. Encouragement of Curiosity and Exploration:

- Childcare professionals encourage children to explore their interests, fostering a sense of curiosity and self-discovery.

- Exploring interests contributes to a positive self-image.

9. Social Skills Development:

- Childcare settings prioritise social skills development, allowing children to build friendships and navigate social interactions.

- Positive peer relationships boost self-esteem.

10. Building Independence:

- Childcare providers help children develop essential life skills such as dressing, feeding and self-care.
- Gaining independence enhances self-worth and pride in personal achievements.

11. Family Involvement:

- Childcare services actively involve families in the child's educational journey, ensuring continuity of support and empowerment.

12. Positive Role Models:

- Childcare providers introduce children to positive role models with disabilities, fostering a sense of possibility and pride.

13. Advocacy for Equal Opportunities:

- Childcare professionals advocate for equal opportunities for children with disabilities, ensuring they have access to inclusive education and play.

14. Celebration of Diversity:

- Childcare settings celebrate diversity by acknowledging and embracing differences among children.
- This promotes a positive attitude towards uniqueness.

In summary, childcare services can significantly contribute to disability empowerment by providing inclusive play and learning, individualised support, early intervention, access to adaptive equipment, communication support, positive reinforcement, sensory activities, encouragement of curiosity, social skills development, building independence, family involvement, exposure to positive role models, advocacy for equal opportunities and the celebration of diversity.

Through these efforts, young children with disabilities can develop a strong sense of self-worth, pride in their accomplishments and a positive self-image that empowers them to thrive as they grow and learn.

9 MENTAL CAPACITY AND DISABILITY EMPOWERMENT

Mental capacity is a fundamental aspect of human autonomy and self-determination and its significance is amplified when it comes to disability empowerment.

The concept of mental capacity encompasses an individual's ability to make informed decisions, understand the consequences of their choices and exercise their own will.

For individuals with disabilities, the journey toward empowerment often involves navigating complex terrain, where varying degrees of mental capacity may intersect with societal expectations and support systems.

Recognising and respecting an individual's mental capacity is essential in promoting their autonomy, self-determination and overall empowerment.

In this context, this discussion explores the intricate relationship between mental capacity and disability empowerment, shedding light on how fostering informed decision-making and self-determination can empower individuals with disabilities to lead more fulfilling lives.

In the United Kingdom, the legal framework concerning mental capacity is primarily governed by the Mental Capacity Act 2005.

This comprehensive legislation provides a structured approach for assessing and making decisions on behalf of individuals who may lack mental capacity to make specific decisions.

The Act is designed to safeguard the rights and best interests of individuals who are deemed to lack capacity due to conditions such as learning disabilities, mental health issues or acquired brain injuries.

Here are some key aspects of the Mental Capacity Act 2005 in the UK:

1. Five Key Principles:

- The Mental Capacity Act is built on five core principles: (a) Presumption of capacity, (b) The right for individuals to make unwise decisions, (c) Best interests as the paramount consideration, (d) Minimal intervention and (e) Least restrictive option.

2. Capacity Assessments:

- The Act outlines a clear process for assessing mental capacity.

- It emphasises that an individual is assumed to have capacity unless proven otherwise.

- Capacity assessments are specific to the decision in question and should consider whether the person can understand, retain, weigh and communicate their decision.

3. Best Interests:

- If an individual is assessed as lacking capacity for a particular decision, the Act stipulates that decisions made on their behalf must be in their best interests.

- The decision-maker should consider the person's past and present wishes, beliefs, values and any available input from family members or care providers.

4. Lasting Power of Attorney (LPA):

- The Mental Capacity Act allows individuals to plan for their future by creating a Lasting Power of Attorney.

- This legal document enables them to appoint someone they trust to make decisions on their behalf if they lose capacity in the future.

5. Court of Protection:

- In situations where disputes arise or complex decisions need to be made, the Court of Protection is responsible for making decisions on behalf of individuals who lack capacity.

- This court ensures that decisions are made in the person's best interests.

7. Supported Decision-Making:

- The Mental Capacity Act encourages the use of supported decision-making, where individuals receive the necessary support and information to make decisions themselves, whenever possible.

The Mental Capacity Act 2005 is a crucial piece of legislation that seeks to balance the protection of vulnerable individuals with disabilities while upholding their autonomy and rights.

It places a strong emphasis on involving individuals in decisions about their care and support, respecting their wishes and feelings and ensuring that any decisions made in their best interests are the least restrictive option.

The Act's principles align with the broader goals of disability empowerment, emphasising the importance of respecting the dignity and autonomy of individuals with disabilities.

The rest of this chapter focuses on principles, capacity assessments and 'best interests'.

How Do the 5 Key Principles Contribute to Disability Empowerment?

The five key principles of the Mental Capacity Act 2005 in the United Kingdom play a significant role in contributing to disability empowerment by providing a legal framework that respects the autonomy and dignity of individuals with disabilities.

Here's how each principle contributes to disability empowerment:

1. Presumption of Capacity:

- **Empowerment Aspect:** This principle starts with the presumption that individuals have the capacity to make decisions unless proven otherwise. It places the emphasis on recognising and respecting an individual's inherent right to make choices.

- **Empowerment Outcome:** By presuming capacity, the principle encourages a culture of empowerment where individuals with disabilities are given the opportunity to express their preferences and participate in decision-making, even if they require support.

2. Right to Make Unwise Decisions:

- **Empowerment Aspect:** This principle recognises that having a disability does not negate a person's right to make decisions, even if those decisions may seem unwise to others.

- **Empowerment Outcome:** It fosters a sense of self-determination and independence by allowing individuals to take calculated risks and learn from their choices, contributing to their personal growth and development.

3. Best Interests as the Paramount Consideration:

- **Empowerment Aspect:** While it's crucial to respect an individual's wishes, this principle ensures that, in cases where capacity is lacking, decisions are made with the person's best interests at heart.

- **Empowerment Outcome:** This principle promotes the empowerment of individuals with disabilities by ensuring that decisions made on their behalf prioritise their welfare and well-being. It prevents decisions that may exploit or harm them.

4. Minimal Intervention:

- **Empowerment Aspect:** The principle of minimal intervention underscores the importance of not overstepping and intervening in an individual's decision-making process unless absolutely necessary.

- **Empowerment Outcome:** It upholds the individual's right to self-determination and independence, allowing them to retain as much control as possible over their lives and choices, even when support is needed.

5. Least Restrictive Option:

- **Empowerment Aspect:** This principle mandates that, when making decisions in someone's best interests, the least restrictive option should be chosen.

- **Empowerment Outcome:** By selecting the least restrictive option, individuals with disabilities are empowered to maintain their freedom and dignity. It ensures that interventions are proportionate and respectful of their rights and preferences.

In summary, the five key principles of the Mental Capacity Act contribute to disability empowerment by establishing a legal framework that preserves an individual's right to make decisions, respects their autonomy and ensures that decisions made on their behalf are in their best interests and as minimally restrictive as possible.

This framework not only safeguards the rights of individuals with disabilities but also promotes their active participation in decision-making, fostering a sense of control, self-worth and empowerment in their lives.

How Do Capacity Assessments Contribute to Disability Empowerment?

Capacity assessments play a crucial role in disability empowerment by ensuring that individuals with disabilities are actively involved in decision-making processes while receiving the necessary support and accommodations. Here's how capacity assessments contribute to disability empowerment:

Respecting Autonomy:

- Capacity assessments begin with the presumption that individuals have the capacity to make decisions unless proven otherwise. This approach respects the autonomy of individuals with disabilities, reinforcing their right to make choices about their lives.

Informed Decision-Making:

- Capacity assessments involve a thorough evaluation of a person's ability to understand, retain, weigh and communicate their decision. This process ensures that individuals receive the information and support needed to make informed choices.

Tailored Support:

- Capacity assessments consider the specific decision in question and the individual's unique needs and preferences. This tailored approach acknowledges that disability does not equate to a lack of capacity across all decisions.

Fostering Independence:

- Capacity assessments aim to determine whether individuals can make decisions independently or with support. When support is necessary, the focus is on empowering individuals to participate actively in decision-making rather than imposing decisions on them.

Reducing Stigmatisation:

- Proper capacity assessments help prevent stigmatisation by avoiding assumptions about an individual's decision-making ability solely based on their disability. This reduces the risk of discrimination and promotes inclusive practices.

Promoting Supported Decision-Making:

- Capacity assessments encourage the use of supported decision-making, where individuals receive the assistance and accommodations required to make choices that align with their values and preferences.

Enhancing Self-Advocacy:

- The assessment process can empower individuals to advocate for themselves, as they become more aware of their decision-making capacity and their rights to express their wishes.

Preventing Unnecessary Interventions:

- By assessing capacity, interventions in individuals' lives are kept to a minimum, ensuring that only necessary actions are taken. This approach reduces the risk of undue interference in their personal affairs.

Balancing Protection and Autonomy:

- Capacity assessments strike a balance between protecting individuals with disabilities from harm and upholding their right to self-determination. This balance is essential for ensuring their well-being while respecting their choices.

Empowering Through Education:

- The capacity assessment process often involves providing individuals with information about their options, risks and benefits. This education empowers them to actively participate in decisions regarding their care, support or treatment.

In summary, capacity assessments contribute to disability empowerment by respecting autonomy, promoting informed decision-making, tailoring support, fostering independence, reducing stigmatisation, supporting self-advocacy, preventing unnecessary interventions, balancing protection and autonomy and empowering individuals through education. These assessments ensure that individuals with disabilities are active participants in their own lives, enabling them to make choices that align with their values, preferences and goals while receiving the necessary support to do so.

How Can the Concept of 'Best Interests' Contribute to Disability Empowerment?

The concept of "best interests" can contribute significantly to disability empowerment by ensuring that decisions made on behalf of individuals with disabilities prioritise their well-being, preferences and rights.

Here's how the concept of "best interests" contributes to disability empowerment:

Balancing Protection and Autonomy:

- The "best interests" principle strikes a balance between protecting individuals with disabilities from harm and respecting their autonomy and self-determination. This balance acknowledges that individuals have the right to make choices that may not align with conventional norms but are still in their best interests.

Individual-Centred Decision-Making:

- The concept of "best interests" requires decision-makers to consider the unique wishes, beliefs, values and preferences of individuals with disabilities when making decisions on their behalf. This individual-centred approach ensures that their voices are heard and respected.

Inclusion of the Person's Perspective:

- Empowering individuals with disabilities often involves actively involving them in the decision-making process. The "best interests" principle encourages the inclusion of the person's perspective and encourages them to express their views about the decisions that affect their lives.

Respecting Dignity and Well-Being:

- Decisions made in a person's best interests prioritise their overall well-being, dignity and quality of life. This approach ensures that individuals are not subjected to decisions that may diminish their self-worth or infringe upon their rights.

Avoiding Arbitrary Decisions:

- The "best interests" principle helps prevent arbitrary decisions made solely based on an individual's disability. Instead, decisions are based on a comprehensive assessment that considers their unique circumstances and needs.

Protection from Exploitation and Harm:

- By requiring decisions to be made in an individual's best interests, this principle safeguards them from potential exploitation, abuse or harm that may result from decisions made without their well-being in mind.

Supporting Informed Choices:

- Decision-makers must provide individuals with disabilities the information and support they need to make informed choices whenever possible. This support empowers them to actively participate in decisions about their care, support or treatment.

Encouraging Least Restrictive Options:

- The "best interests" principle promotes the selection of the least restrictive options when making decisions. This ensures that individuals have the opportunity to maintain their freedom and independence to the greatest extent possible.

Adaptation to Changing Circumstances:

- "Best interests" assessments are dynamic and adaptable, taking into account changing circumstances and the evolving wishes and needs of individuals with disabilities. This flexibility supports their ongoing empowerment.

Legal Safeguards:

- Legal frameworks, such as the Mental Capacity Act 2005 in the UK, provide clear guidelines for assessing and determining a person's best interests. These legal safeguards ensure that the principle is applied consistently and transparently.

In summary, the concept of "best interests" contributes to disability empowerment by promoting a balanced approach that respects autonomy while safeguarding individuals with disabilities from harm.

It ensures that decisions are individual-centred, based on their unique needs and preferences and that they actively participate in the decision-making process.

This approach empowers individuals with disabilities to lead more self-determined lives while receiving the support and protection they may need.

Personal Judgement and Disability Empowerment

Interpretation of the Mental Capacity Act (MCA) and its Code of Practice can rely on personal judgment, to a certain extent.

The MCA and its accompanying Code provide a legal framework and guidance for assessing and making decisions on behalf of individuals who may lack capacity.

However, due to the complex and nuanced nature of capacity assessments and decision-making, there is often a degree of subjectivity involved.

Here's how personal judgment comes into play:

1. **Assessing Capacity:** The MCA outlines the criteria for assessing mental capacity, including a person's ability to understand, retain, weigh and communicate their decision. Interpreting these criteria can involve some subjectivity, as professionals must use their judgment to determine whether an individual meets these criteria for a specific decision.

2. **Best Interests Determination:** When making decisions in someone's best interests, the MCA requires decision-makers to consider various factors, including the person's past and present wishes, beliefs, values and any available input from family members or care providers. This process often requires subjective judgment in weighing and prioritising these factors.

3. **Least Restrictive Option:** The principle of choosing the least restrictive option involves considering what interventions or actions are necessary while minimising the impact on the individual's rights and freedoms. This determination often relies on personal judgment to strike a balance.

4. **Supported Decision-Making:** The MCA encourages supported decision-making, where individuals receive the assistance they need to make decisions themselves. The extent and nature of this support can vary based on individual circumstances, requiring personal judgment to tailor the support effectively.

5. **Court of Protection:** In complex cases or disputes, the Court of Protection may be involved in making decisions on behalf of individuals who lack capacity.

Judges and legal professionals exercise their judgment to apply the law and assess best interests in these situations.

While personal judgment plays a role in interpreting and applying the MCA, it's crucial to note that the Act provides clear legal principles and procedural safeguards to guide decision-makers and minimise the risk of arbitrary or biased decisions.

Additionally, decisions made under the MCA are subject to legal oversight and can be challenged if they are deemed to be inconsistent with the law or the individual's best interests.

The aim is to ensure transparency, fairness and the protection of the rights and well-being of individuals with disabilities.

Interpretation and the Effects on Disability Empowerment

The interpretation of the Mental Capacity Act (MCA) and its Code of Practice can significantly affect disability empowerment, both positively and negatively, depending on how it is applied.

Here's how the interpretation of the MCA can impact disability empowerment:

Positive Impact on Disability Empowerment:

1. **Respecting Autonomy:** A broad and inclusive interpretation of the MCA's criteria for assessing capacity can promote disability empowerment by respecting individuals' autonomy and their right to make decisions, even if those decisions are unconventional or unwise in the eyes of others. This

approach empowers individuals to express their preferences and actively participate in decisions about their lives.

2. **Individual-Centred Approach:** A person-centred and individualised interpretation of the MCA supports disability empowerment by acknowledging that each person with a disability is unique. It ensures that decisions are tailored to their specific needs, preferences and circumstances, promoting their self-determination.

3. **Supported Decision-Making:** An interpretation of the MCA that strongly encourages and facilitates supported decision-making empowers individuals with disabilities by providing them with the necessary assistance to make choices aligned with their values. This approach promotes their active participation in decisions affecting their lives.

4. **Minimising Restrictiveness:** Interpreting the MCA's principle of choosing the least restrictive option with flexibility can empower individuals by allowing them to retain as much freedom and independence as possible. This approach helps prevent unnecessary restrictions on their rights and choices.

Negative Impact on Disability Empowerment:

1. **Overly Restrictive Interpretation:** An overly cautious or restrictive interpretation of the MCA can have a negative impact on disability empowerment by limiting individuals' autonomy. It may result in decisions that unnecessarily curtail their rights and choices, undermining their sense of self-determination.

2. **Ignoring Individuality:** Failing to take an individualised approach to capacity assessments and decision-making can disempower individuals with disabilities by treating them as a homogeneous group rather than recognising their unique needs, preferences and capacities.

3. **Underestimating Capacity:** If professionals consistently underestimate an individual's capacity based solely on their disability, it can lead to a lack of respect for their autonomy and decision-making abilities. This undermines their empowerment and can perpetuate stereotypes.

4. **Limited Support:** A lack of emphasis on supported decision-making in interpretation and practice can hinder disability empowerment. Without adequate support, individuals may struggle to assert their choices and preferences effectively.

In summary, the interpretation of the Mental Capacity Act can significantly affect disability empowerment. A thoughtful and person-centred interpretation that upholds the principles of autonomy, individuality and supported decision-making can enhance empowerment. Conversely, an interpretation that is overly restrictive, disregards individuality, or underestimates capacity may hinder disability empowerment by limiting individuals' rights and choices. It is essential for professionals and decision-makers to strike a balance that respects the rights and well-being of individuals with disabilities while providing necessary support and safeguards.

10 SUMMARY AND CONCLUSIONS

In the journey toward disability empowerment, we have explored the intricate web of principles, practices and legal frameworks that underpin the rights and autonomy of individuals with disabilities.

This final chapter serves as a culmination of our exploration, summarising the key insights and conclusions drawn from the discussions.

1. Embracing Individuality and Personalisation:

- Disability empowerment thrives when we recognise and celebrate the uniqueness of each person with a disability.

- Tailoring support and accommodations to their specific needs, preferences and goals fosters a sense of empowerment and self-determination.

2. Autonomy and Informed Decision-Making:

- The cornerstone of empowerment is respecting individuals' right to make choices about their lives.

- Empowering practices involve providing the necessary information and support for informed decision-making while honouring their autonomy.

3. Self-Determination:

- Empowerment is achieved when individuals actively participate in decisions about their care, support and life goals.

- Self-determination allows them to assert their preferences, set goals and take charge of their destinies.

4. Advocacy and Equal Access:

- Empowerment extends beyond individual experiences; it encompasses advocating for the rights of people with disabilities at a societal level.

- Ensuring equal access to services, employment, education and challenging discrimination are integral aspects of disability empowerment.

5. Skill-Building:

- Providing individuals with disabilities the skills and tools they need to live independently enhances their empowerment.

- Skills like communication, problem-solving and self-advocacy equip them to navigate life's challenges confidently.

6. Support Networks:

- Building and nurturing support networks, both formal and informal, is essential.

- Peer support groups, community resources and social

services provide a vital safety net and a sense of belonging.

7. Accessibility and Inclusion:

- True empowerment requires accessible environments and inclusive communities where individuals with disabilities can fully participate and engage.

- Removing physical and societal barriers is a collective responsibility.

8. Fostering a Positive Self-Image:

- Challenging stereotypes and promoting a positive self-image and self-esteem are central to empowerment.

- Recognising and valuing one's abilities and worth is foundational to leading a fulfilling life.

9. Monitoring and Evaluation:

- Regularly assessing the effectiveness of care services and making adjustments as needed is crucial.

- This ensures that care plans remain aligned with individuals' evolving needs and goals.

10. Mental Capacity and Best Interests:

- The Mental Capacity Act provides a legal framework that respects the autonomy and dignity of individuals with disabilities.

- Decision-makers must strike a balance between protection and empowerment, always considering the best interests of the individual.

11. The Role of Advocacy:

- Advocacy efforts, whether at an individual or systemic level, are indispensable in promoting and protecting the rights and empowerment of individuals with disabilities.

12. The Importance of Education:

- Educating individuals with disabilities about their rights and equipping them with the knowledge and skills to advocate for themselves is pivotal in empowerment.

13. Celebrating Progress and Acknowledging Challenges:

- While we have made significant strides in disability empowerment, challenges persist.

- Recognising these challenges is essential for continued progress.

In conclusion, disability empowerment is a multifaceted journey that encompasses recognising the value of every individual, upholding their rights and autonomy and challenging barriers and stereotypes.

It requires a collective effort from individuals, communities, organisations and policymakers to create a world where disability is not a limitation but a diverse aspect of the human experience.

As we conclude this exploration, let us carry forward the principles and practices of disability empowerment, ensuring that every person, regardless of their abilities, can thrive and lead a life of dignity, choice and fulfilment.

ABOUT THE AUTHOR

Susan Rogers (HSC Training Link) has been providing resources for the health and social care sector since 2004.